Color Atlas of
Brain Disorders
in the Newborn

L.S. de Vries • *L.M.S. Dubowitz*
V. Dubowitz • *J.M. Pennock*

Royal Postgraduate Medical School
Hammersmith Hospital
London

Year Book Medical Publishers Inc.

Year Book Medical Publishers Inc.
200 North LaSalle Street
Chicago, Illinois 60601, USA

First Published by Wolfe Medical Publications Ltd,
2-16 Torrington Place, London WC1E 7LT, UK
Printed by W.S. Cowell Ltd, Ipswich, England

First edition, 1990

ISBN 0-8151-2964-5

Library of Congress Cataloging-in-Publication Data

A color atlas of brain disorders in the newborn/L.S. deVries . . . [et al.]
    p.   cm.
    Includes bibliographical references.
    ISBN 0-8151-2964-5
    1. Brain—Diseases—Magnetic resonance imaging—Atlases.
2. Brain—Diseases—Diagnosis—Atlases. 3. Infants (newborn)—
—Diseases—Diagnosis—Atlases. I. DeVries, L.S.
    [DNLM: 1. Brain Diseases—in infancy & childhood—atlases.
2. Brain Diseases—pathology—atlases. 3. Infant, Newborn,
Diseases—atlases. WS 17 C718]
RJ290.5.C65 1990
618.92′8047548′0222—dc20
DNLM/DLC   89-24886
for Library of Congress   CIP

Contents

Acknowledgements   4

Introduction   5

1. Principles of Magnetic Resonance Imaging   19

2. Intraventricular and Periventricular Haemorrhage   29

3. Leukomalacia   69

4. Cerebral Artery Infarction   135

5. Haemorrhagic and Ischaemic Lesions of Antenatal Origin   144

6. Hypoxic Ischaemic Encephalopathy in the Full Term Infant   168

MRI: Glossary, References and Further Reading   194

Index   195

Acknowledgements

We are grateful to a large number of people for their expertise and advice in the preparation of this Atlas. Jonathan Wigglesworth provided all the neuropathological backup, and Graeme Bydder the extensive interpretation on magnetic resonance imaging, both of which formed a vital core of the study. Rivka Regev contributed substantially to the clinical assessment of the babies, combining her clinical acumen with a remarkable empathy.

The comprehensive physiological studies, which included continuous electroencephalogram monitoring by John Connell and Rowena Oozeer, auditory brainstem responses by Sana Lary, visual evoked responses by Joan Mushin, and Doppler blood flow velocities by Frances Cowan and intracranial pressure measurements by Anthony Kaiser greatly helped to extend the scope of the Atlas. We are grateful to the photographic and medical art department, and David Hawtin in particular, for the superb clinical photography, and to the CT Scanner unit for the CT imaging. We are also grateful to the nursing staff of the Neonatal unit and the Childrens' Outpatient department, who were always tolerant and extremely helpful; to the infants and their parents for their cooperation; and to the clinicians who referred their patients to us.

We also appreciate the efforts of the editorial staff of Wolfe Medical, and especially those of Nigel Balmforth and latterly Paul Bennett, in guiding this Atlas through its somewhat interrupted labour pangs and delivery.

We are grateful to the Medical Research Council, the Department of Health especially Gordon Higson, and Action Research for the Crippled Child, for financial support.

Introduction

Haemorrhagic and ischaemic lesions of the brain during the perinatal period are a major cause of mortality and morbidity in the preterm and full term infant. The association between these lesions and the development of cerebral palsy has been recognised for several decades, but until recently these lesions could only be diagnosed at autopsy. The advent of X-ray computed tomography (CT) scanning and then ultrasound (US) imaging of the newborn brain made the diagnosis of brain lesions possible during life.

Haemorrhages in the brain were diagnosed in newborn infants by CT scanning in the late 1970s, but this technique was impractical for routine use as it involved the transfer of the infant from the neonatal unit to the scanner. On the other hand ultrasound equipment could be brought to the bedside; it was completely safe and non-invasive and repeated scanning could be done without any disturbance to the infant or interruption to her or his management. This opened the way not only for identifying haemorrhagic and ischaemic lesions of the newborn brain but also for following their evolution and resolution and correlating other modalities of assessment with the presence of these lesions.

The purpose of this atlas is to illustrate the way in which ultrasound, together with clinical assessment, electrophysiological studies, X-ray computed tomography and magnetic resonance imaging (MRI) has helped in the diagnosis, assessment and prognostication of these lesions.

Ultrasound Imaging

The early linear array machines with 3.5 and 5 MHz transducers were capable of detecting haemorrhage which produced areas of increased echogenicity. The standard cuts were transverse (horizontal) through the temporal bone. On these images the presence or absence of haemorrhage could be identified (1).

With improvement in the equipment, scanning through the anterior fontanelle became possible, allowing not only the diagnosis of haemorrhage but a better appreciation of the size of the lesion

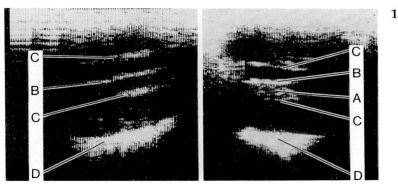

1

Comparison of normal high axial scan (left) with a scan showing IVH in the lateral ventricle (A). Note the falx (B), lateral wall of lateral ventricle (C) and skull echo (D).

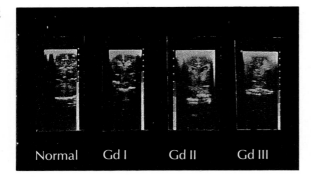

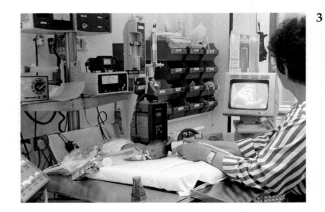

and of the lateral ventricles. However, the field visualised with the linear scanner was very narrow and the full extent of the lesions could not be appreciated (2)

The introduction of sector scanners with 5 and 7.5 MHz transducers (3) led to a marked improvement in resolution and also a wider field of view through the anterior fontanelle, with the ability

not only to identify but also to grade lesions.

The angles of the standard cuts through the anterior fontanelle are shown in the mid-coronal plane, angling the scan head forwards through the frontal lobes and backwards towards the occipital lobes (4). Longitudinal sections in the sagittal and parasagittal planes parallel to the midline are shown in 5.

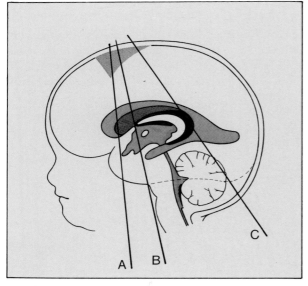

A = scan through frontal horn
B = scan through foramen of Monro
C = scan through trigone

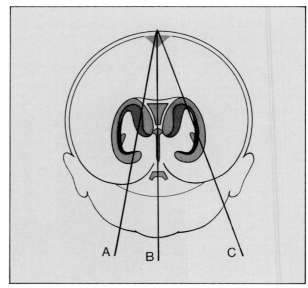

A = scan through head of caudate nucleus
B = scan through the midline
C = scan through body of lateral ventricle

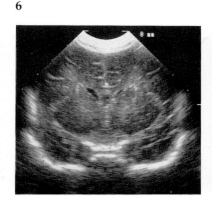
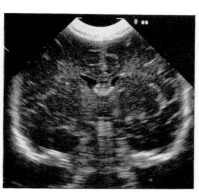
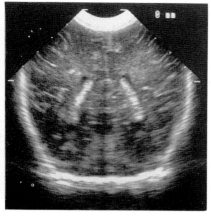

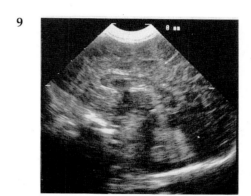
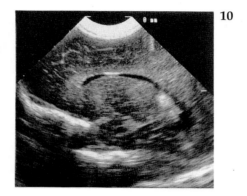

The normal appearances in the coronal cuts are shown in **6**, **7** and **8**, the sagittal and parasagittal views in **9** and **10**. The coronal ultrasound images are displayed with the right side of the child's brain on the right of the image. In the sagittal and parasagittal views the anterior horns are on the left of the picture and the posterior horns on the right.

With these standard sections it was possible to localise and grade haemorrhage accurately. Lesions in the periventricular areas such as periventricular leukomalacia, and lesions further out in the brain parenchyma, such as subcortical leukomalacia and infarction, could also be recognised.

Cumulative data on the occurrence and evolution of haemorrhagic and ischaemic lesions have produced useful information on the timing of these lesions during the postnatal period. Haemorrhages are rarely present at birth; most occur in the first 72 hours, and only a few after this period.

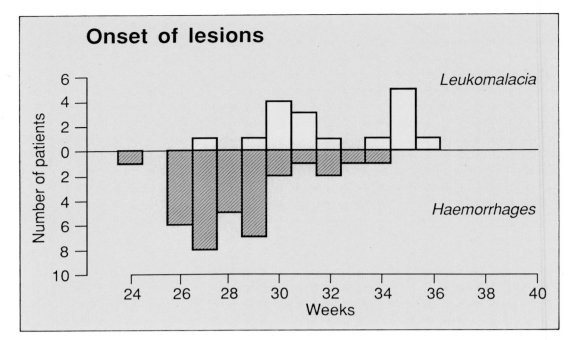

The relationship of different gestational age to haemorrhagic and ischaemic lesions can also be demonstrated (**11**). The value of repeated ultrasound scanning is summarised below.

Value of Ultrasound

- diagnosis of lesion
- type and site of lesion
- timing of lesion
- natural evolution
- response to treatment
- effect on clinical signs
- effect on physiological events

Clinical Evaluation

When intraventricular haemorrhage was first recognised by Papile and her colleagues with CT scanning, they found a remarkably high incidence (approximately 50%) in preterm infants under 1500 grams. They noted that a large proportion of the infants appeared to be clinically 'silent' or normal. One possible explanation for this may have been the inadequacy of the clinical methods used for the evaluation of the nervous system of the preterm infant.

One of our main objectives was to evolve a system for the neurological assessment of the newborn infant which was sensitive, simple and reliable, as well as effective for the preterm and fullterm infant. It was also necessary to be able to monitor the progress of an individual infant and follow a large number of individual signs.

A system was evolved which integrated a selection of items reflecting posture, tone, primitive reflexes and neurobehavioural responses. These were tabulated in a proforma with a scoring system for individual signs of five grades, based on increasing response of that particular sign. Detailed instruction on the evaluation of each sign was also introduced in the proforma which could be used as a record for each individual examination. The documentation of individual items could be done directly on the proforma sheet by circling each individual sign (**12** and **13**).

By using a separate sheet for sequential examinations of the same infant, a comprehensive record of maturation in the normal 'optimal' premature infant, or the progress in an ill infant, could be documented. The evolution and resolution of deviant neurological signs could also be accurately and objectively recorded. Thus a comparison could be made of the neurological status of the preterm infant reaching 40 weeks postmenstrual age (PMA) with that of the newborn full term infant at 40 weeks gestation.

NAME	D.O.B./TIME	WEIGHT	E.D.D. L.N.M.P.	E.D.D. U/snd.	STATES	STATE	COMMENT	ASYMMETRY
HOSP. NO.	DATE OF EXAM	HEIGHT			1. Deep sleep, no movement, regular breathing. 2. Light sleep, eyes shut, some movement. 3. Dozing, eyes opening and closing. 4. Awake, eyes open, minimal movement. 5. Wide awake, vigorous movement. 6. Crying.			
RACE SEX	AGE	HEAD CIRC.	GESTATIONAL ASSESSMENT	SCORE WEEKS				

HABITUATION (⩽state 3)

LIGHT
Repetitive flashlight stimuli (10) with 5 sec. gap.
Shutdown = 2 consecutive negative responses

| No response | A. Blink response to first stimulus only. B. Tonic blink response. C. Variable response. | A. Shutdown of movement but blink persists 2-5 stimuli. B. Complete shutdown 2-5 stimuli. | A. Shutdown of movement but blink persists 6-10 stimuli. B. Complete shutdown 6-10 stimuli. | A. Equal response to 10 stimuli. B. Infant comes to fully alert state. C. Startles + major responses throughout. |

RATTLE
Repetitive stimuli (10) with 5 sec. gap.

| No response | A. Slight movement to first stimulus. B. Variable response. | Startle or movement 2-5 stimuli, then shutdown | Startle or movement 6-10 stimuli, then shutdown | A. B. Grading as above C. |

MOVEMENT & TONE
Undress infant

POSTURE *
(At rest — predominant)

(hips abducted)   (hips adducted)

Abnormal postures:
A. Opisthotonus.
B. Unusual leg extension.
C. Asymm. tonic neck reflex

ARM RECOIL
Infant supine. Take both hands, extend parallel to the body; hold approx. 2 secs. and release.

| No flexion within 5 sec. | Partial flexion at elbow >100° within 4-5 sec. | Arms flex at elbow to <100° within 2-3 sec. | Sudden jerky flexion at elbow immediately after release to <60° | Difficult to extend; arm snaps back forcefully |

ARM TRACTION
Infant supine; head midline; grasp wrist, slowly pull arm to vertical. Angle of arm scored and resistance noted at moment infant is initially lifted off and watched until shoulder off mattress. Do other arm.

| Arm remains fully extended | Weak flexion maintained only momentarily | Arm flexed at elbow to 140° and maintained 5 sec. | Arm flexed at approx. 100° and maintained | Strong flexion of arm <100° and maintained |

LEG RECOIL
First flex hips for 5 secs. then extend both legs of infant by traction on ankles; hold down on the bed for 2 secs. and release.

| No flexion within 5 sec. | Incomplete flexion of hips within 5 sec. | Complete flexion within 5 sec. | Instantaneous complete flexion | Legs cannot be extended; snap back forcefully |

LEG TRACTION
Infant supine. Grasp leg near ankle and slowly pull toward vertical until buttocks 1-2" off. Note resistance at knee and score angle. Do other leg.

| No flexion | Partial flexion, rapidly lost | Knee flexion 140-160° and maintained | Knee flexion 100-140° and maintained | Strong resistance; flexion <100° |

POPLITEAL ANGLE
Infant supine. Approximate knee and thigh to abdomen; extend leg by gentle pressure with index finger behind ankle

| 180-160° | 150-140° | 130-120° | 110-90° | <90° |

HEAD CONTROL (post. neck m.)
Grasp infant by shoulders and raise to sitting position; allow head to fall forward; wait 30 sec.

| No attempt to raise head | Unsuccessful attempt to raise head upright | Head raised smoothly to upright in 30 sec. but not maintained. | Head raised smoothly to upright in 30 sec. and maintained | Head cannot be flexed forward |

HEAD CONTROL (ant. neck m.)
Allow head to fall backward as you hold shoulders; wait 30 secs.

| Grading as above | Grading as above | Grading as above | Grading as above | |

HEAD LAG *
Pull infant toward sitting posture by traction on both wrists. Also note arm flexion.

VENTRAL SUSPENSION *
Hold infant in ventral suspension; observe curvature of back, flexion of limbs and relation of head to trunk.

HEAD RAISING IN PRONE POSITION
Infant in prone position with head in midline.

| No response | Rolls head to one side | Weak effort to raise head and turns raised head to one side | Infant lifts head, nose and chin off | Strong prolonged head lifting |

ARM RELEASE IN PRONE POSITION
Head in midline. Infant in prone position; arms extended alongside body with palms up.

| No effort | Some effort and wriggling | Flexion effort but neither wrist brought to nipple level | One or both wrists brought at least to nipple level without excessive body movement | Strong body movement with both wrists brought to face, or 'press-ups' |

SPONTANEOUS BODY MOVEMENT
during examination (supine). If no spont. movement try to induce by cutaneous stimulation.

| None or minimal Induced | A. Sluggish. B. Random, incoordinated. C. Mainly stretching. | Smooth movements alternating with random, stretching, athetoid or jerky. | Smooth alternating movements of arms and legs with medium speed and intensity | Mainly: A. Jerky movement. B. Athetoid movement. C. Other abnormal movement. | 1 2 |

TREMORS   Mark: Fast (>6/sec.) or Slow (<6/sec.)

| No tremor | Tremors only in state 5-6 | Tremors only in sleep or after Moro and startles | Some tremors in state 4 | Tremulousness in all states |

STARTLES

| No startles | Startles to sudden noise, Moro, bang on table only | Occasional spontaneous startle | 2-5 spontaneous startles | 6 + spontaneous startles |

ABNORMAL MOVEMENT OR POSTURE

| No abnormal movement | A. Hands clenched but open intermittently. B. Hands do not open with Moro. | A. Some mouthing movement. B. Intermittent adducted thumb | A. Persistently adducted thumb. B. Hands clenched all the time. | A. Continuous mouthing movement. B. Abnormal toe posture. C. Abnormal finger posture. D. Convulsive movement. |

9

| | | | | | | STATE | COMMENT | ASYMMETRY |

REFLEXES

						STATE	COMMENT	ASYMMETRY
TENDON REFLEXES Biceps jerk Knee jerk Ankle jerk	Absent		Present	Exaggerated	Clonus			
PALMAR GRASP Head in midline. Put index finger from ulnar side into hand and gently press palmar surface. Never touch dorsal side of hand.	Absent	Short, weak flexion	Medium strength and sustained flexion for several secs.	Strong flexion; contraction spreads to forearm	Very strong grasp. Infant easily lifts off couch			
	R L	R L	R L	R L	R L			
PLANTAR GRASP Press the thumb against the ball of the infants foot.	No response	Partial plantar flexion of toes.	Toes curl around examiners finger.					
	R L	R L	R L					
ROOTING Infant supine, head midline. Touch each corner of the mouth in turn (stroke laterally).	No response	A. Partial weak head turn but no mouth opening. B. Mouth opening, no head turn.	Mouth opening on stimulated side with partial head turning	Full head turning with or without mouth opening	Mouth opening with very jerky head turning			
SUCKING Infant supine; place index finger (pad towards palate) in infant's mouth; judge power of sucking movement after 5 sec.	No attempt	Weak sucking movement: A. Regular. B. Irregular.	Strong sucking movement, poor stripping: A. Regular. B. Irregular.	Strong regular sucking movement with continuing sequence of 5 movements. Good stripping.	Clenching but no regular sucking.			
WALKING (state 4, 5) Hold infant upright, feet touching bed, neck held straight with fingers.	Absent		Some effort but not continuous with both legs	At least 2 steps with both legs	A. Stork posture; no movement. B. Automatic walking.			
PLACING Lift infant in an upright position and allow dorsum of foot to touch protruding edge of a flat surface.	No response	Dorsiflexion of ankle only	Full placing response with flexion of hip and knee and placing sole of foot on surface.					
	R L	R L	R L					
MORO One hand supports infant's head in midline, the other his back. Raise infant to 45° and when infant is relaxed let his head fall through 10°. Note if jerky. Repeat 3 times.	No response, or opening of hands only	Full abduction at the shoulder and extension of the arm	Full abduction but only delayed or partial adduction	Partial abduction at shoulder and extension of arms followed by smooth adduction	A. No abduction or adduction; extension only. B. Marked adduction only. A. Abd>Add B. Abd=Add C. Abd<Add	J	S	

NEUROBEHAVIOURAL ITEMS

						STATE	COMMENT	ASYMMETRY
EYE APPEARANCES	Sunset sign Nerve palsy	Transient nystagmus. Strabismus. Transient roving eye movement.	Does not open eyes	Normal conjugate eye movement	A. Persistent nystagmus. B. Frequent roving movement C. Frequent rapid blinks.			
AUDITORY ORIENTATION (state 3, 4) To rattle. (Note presence of startle.)	A. No reaction. B. Auditory startle but no true orientation.	Brightens and stills; may turn toward stimuli with eyes closed	Alerting and shifting of eyes; head may or may not turn to source	Alerting; prolonged head turns to stimulus; search with eyes	Turning and alerting to stimulus each time on both sides		S	
VISUAL ORIENTATION (state 4) To red woollen ball	Does not focus or follow stimulus	Stills; focuses on stimulus; may follow 30° jerkily; does not find stimulus again spontaneously	Follows 30-60° horizontally; may lose stimulus but finds it again. Brief vertical glance	Follows with eyes and head horizontally and to some extent vertically, with frowning	Sustained fixation; follows vertically, horizonally, and in circle			
ALERTNESS/ RESPONSIVENESS Do not score appearance but responsiveness to visual stimulation.	Inattentive; rarely or never responds to direct stimulation	When alert, periods rather brief; rather variable response to orientation	When alert, alertness moderately sustained; may use stimulus to come to alert state	Sustained alertness; orientation frequent; reliable to visual stimuli.	Continuous alertness, which does not seem to tire, to visual stimuli.			
DEFENSIVE REACTION A cloth or hand is placed over the infant's face to partially occlude the nasal airway.	No response	A. General quietening. B. Non-specific activity with long latency.	Rooting; lateral neck turning; possibly neck stretching.	Swipes with arm	Swipes with arm with rather violent body movement			
PEAK OF EXCITEMENT	Low level arousal to all stimuli; never > state 3	Infant reaches state 4-5 briefly but predominantly in lower states	Infant predominantly state 4 or 5; may reach state 6 after stimulation but returns spontaneously to lower state	Infant reaches state 6 but can be consoled relatively easily	A. Mainly state 6. Difficult to console, if at all. B. Mainly state 4-5 but if reaches state 6 cannot be consoled.			
IRRITABILITY (states 3, 4, 5) Aversive stimuli: Uncover Ventral susp. Undress Moro Pull to sit Walking reflex Prone	No irritable crying to any of the stimuli	Cries to 1-2 stimuli	Cries to 3-4 stimuli	Cries to 5-6 stimuli	Cries to all stimuli			
CONSOLABILITY (state 6)	Never above state 5 during examination, therefore not needed	Consoling not needed. Consoles spontaneously	Consoled by talking, hand on belly or wrapping up	Consoled by picking up and holding; may need finger in mouth	Not consolable			
CRY	No cry at all	Only whimpering cry	Cries to stimuli but normal pitch	Lusty cry to offensive stimuli; normal pitch	High-pitched cry, often continuous			

NOTES ✳ If asymmetrical or atypical, draw in on nearest figure. Record any abnormal signs (e.g. facial palsy, contractures, etc.). Draw if possible.

CHECK LIST OF ABNORMAL SIGNS

Head and trunk control	Orientation & alertness
Limb tone	Irritability
Motility	Consolability
Reflexes	Deviant sign

Modified from *The Neurological Assessment of the Preterm and Full-term Newborn Infant*, by Lilly and Victor Dubowitz

© 1981 Spastics International Medical Publications, 5A Netherhall Gardens, London NW3 5RN.

Record time after feed:

EXAMINER:

This comparison revealed a number of differences, including some in tone and posture. Differences between a full term infant during the first few days of life (**14**, **16** and **18**) and an infant born at 28 weeks gestation reaching 40 weeks PMA (**15**, **17** and **19**) are illustrated, in the supine position (**14** and **15**) and in ventral suspension (**16** and **17**). The difference in resistance to arm traction is illustrated in **18** and **19**. Thus it was possible to define a norm in preterm infants at 40 weeks postmenstrual age.

14

15
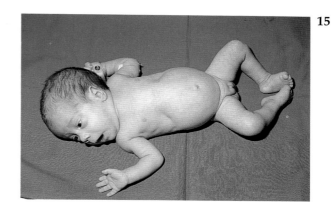

16
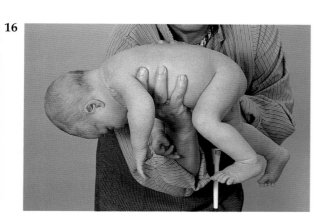

17
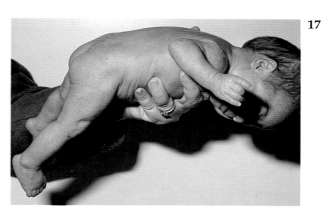

18
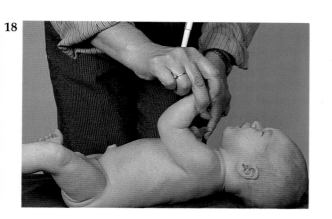

19
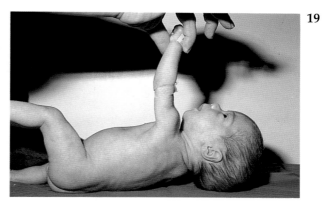

From this baseline, abnormal neurological signs in the individual ill infant could be recognised. These could take the form of abnormal maturation in relation to gestational age, which could be either delayed, 'accelerated' or deviant. Delayed development is illustrated in relation to development of poor posture of the head and trunk in ventral suspension (20), and poor head control when pulled to sit. Accelerated maturation may take the form of 'too good' head control in ventral suspension in an infant of 32 weeks PMA (21), due to excessive extensor tone.

20
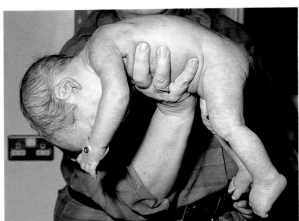

21
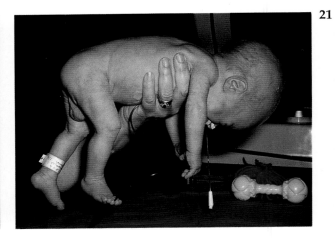

22
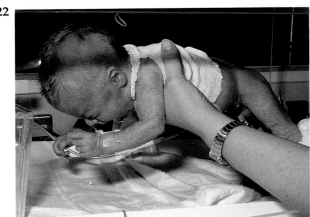

23
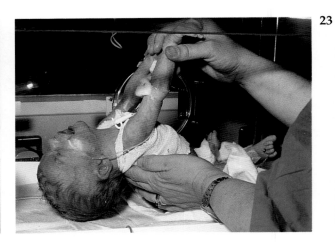

Aberrant Signs

- differential head control
- arm flexion > leg flexion
- tight popliteal angle
- frequent tremors and startles
- asymmetries
- absent plantar grasp
- abnormal Moro
- abnormal finger or toe posture
- irritability

A number of aberrant signs can also be identified. Those of particular interest are summarised in the table (left).

Abnormal tone patterns showing differential head control are illustrated in **22** and **23**. Note increased extensor tone of the trunk and neck muscles in ventral suspension (**22**) and poor head control when pulled to sit (**23**).

Abnormal tone pattern consisting of marked flexor tone in the arm in association with increased extensor tone in the limbs is shown in **24**.

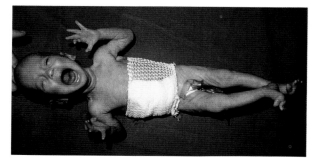

Also note the abnormal toe postures (spontaneous Babinski) and the abnormal finger posture, with flexion of thumb and index finger. The infant is also extremely irritable.

The detection of aberrant signs in individual infants and their correlation with the presence of haemorrhagic and ischaemic lesions on ultrasound examination have enabled us to recognise several

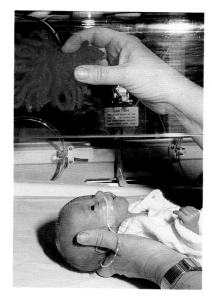

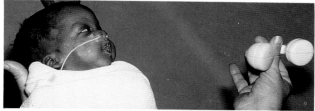

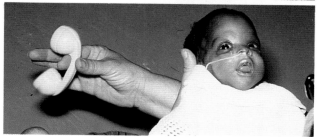

patterns of clinical signs. These are distinctive for a particular lesion and can be extremely useful in the clinical diagnosis of haemorrhagic and ischaemic lesions. Their persistence or/and resolution may also give a better basis for prognosis.

Assessment of hearing and vision forms part of the routine clinical examination and can be readily elicited by simple bedside testing. Visual tracking in the full term as well as preterm infant can be accurately assessed with a red woollen ball held at a distance of approximately 20cm (**25**).

Hearing is assessed with a simple plastic rattle which produces a white noise of 60–80 dB intensity. This is as sensitive as more sophisticated tools and will pick up both unilateral and bilateral hearing loss of 60 dB. The infant illustrated in **26** showed a brisk response on the left to the rattle but not on the right. Electrophysiological testing confirmed a hearing threshold of 80 dB on the left but a normal hearing threshold of 40 dB on the right.

In addition to reflecting the state of the nervous system, visual and auditory responses may also help to pinpoint an isolated visual or auditory deficit. If suspected on clinical assessment, confirmation can be obtained by appropriate electrophysiological evaluation of the visual and auditory pathways.

Electrophysiology

Auditory Brainstem Evoked Responses (ABR):
Measurement of ABR is a well standardised technique which is easy to perform in newborn infants (**27**). It involves providing an auditory stimulus via an earphone in the form of high frequency clicks, and recording the response via electrodes placed on the mastoid and vertex.

The fully mature response has six detectable waves (**28**), and information on different parts of the auditory pathway can be obtained by calculating the latency and amplitude of these waves and the intervals between them. The I–V latency is known as brainstem transmission time. **29** illustrates the maturation of these wave forms with gestational age. Note that latencies shorten and amplitude increases. ABR is of value in detecting both hearing difficulty and brainstem dysfunction.

27

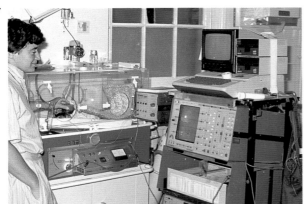

28

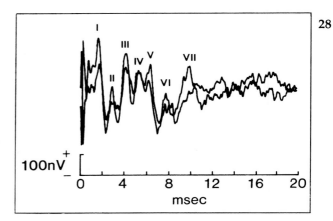

29

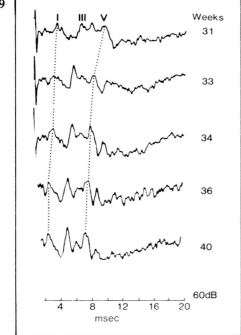

30

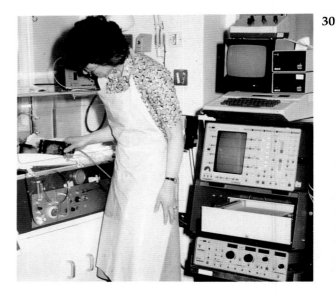

Visual Evoked Responses (VER) are obtained by using an appropriate visual stimulus such as a stroboscope or, preferably, diodes emitting red light (**30**). The latter can penetrate the closed eyelids of the infant, and a record of the response from the occipital cortex can be obtained. The mature trace shows a series of negative and positive waves.

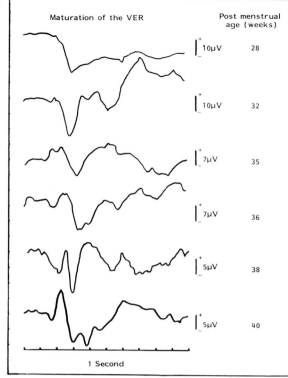

Maturation of the VER

Post menstrual age (weeks)

	Post menstrual age (weeks)
10μV	28
10μV	32
7μV	35
7μV	36
5μV	38
5μV	40

1 Second

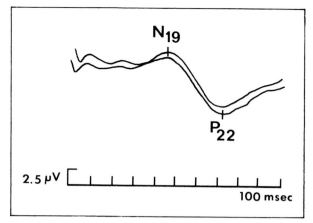

N₁₉

P₂₂

2.5 μV

100 msec

During early gestation the response consists of a negative wave only, but by 32–34 weeks a positive wave preceding the negative wave appears. The maturation of this response with gestational age (negativity recorded downwards) is given in **31**. VER is a sensitive test for the integrity of the visual pathways and the effect of lesions in the brain on these pathways. VER also plays an important part in verifying cortical blindness.

Somatosensory Evoked Responses (SER): Following electrical stimulation of the median or tibial nerve, a response is recorded from the contralateral parietal cortex. It is of potential value in documenting the integrity of the sensory tracts of the nervous system. We have not used this technique routinely on our infants. Experience and data with this method are increasing, and SER have a strong predictive value for neurodevelopmental outcome. A normal recording is shown in **32**.

Electroencephalography (EEG): With the introduction of the Oxford Medilog four-channel recorder it became practical to record continuous EEG activity in sick newborn infants without any distress to the infant or interruption to its intensive care or management (**33**). EEG recordings from 28 weeks gestation to term have been made to determine the process of maturation. Initially a very discontinuous pattern with intermittent bursts of activity is seen. This pattern becomes predominantly continuous, with only short periods of inactivity during quiet sleep, at term (**34**). By dividing 24 hour periods of recording into five minute epochs in optimal preterm and term infants, it has been possible to quantify the proportion of continuity and discontinuity of the tracings in relation to gestation, and to produce graphs of normal values (**35**).

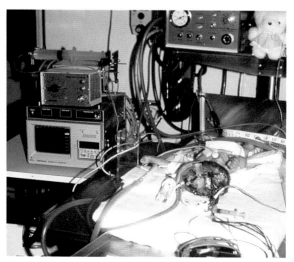

34

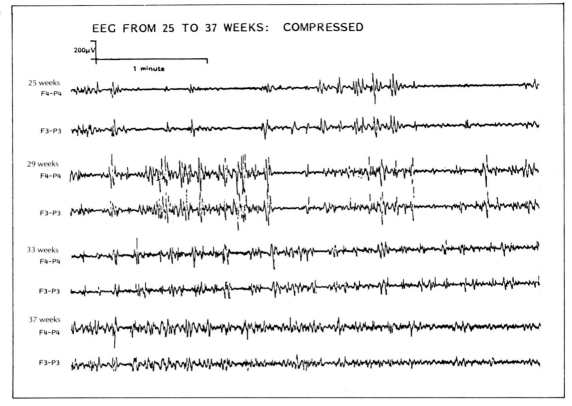

EEG FROM 25 TO 37 WEEKS: COMPRESSED

200μV

1 minute

25 weeks
F4-P4

F3-P3

29 weeks
F4-P4

F3-P3

33 weeks
F4-P4

F3-P3

37 weeks
F4-P4

F3-P3

35

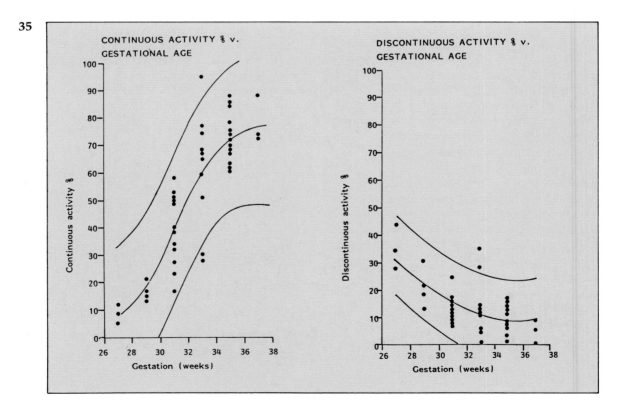

CONTINUOUS ACTIVITY % v.
GESTATIONAL AGE

DISCONTINUOUS ACTIVITY % v.
GESTATIONAL AGE

Continuous activity %

Gestation (weeks)

Discontinuous activity %

Gestation (weeks)

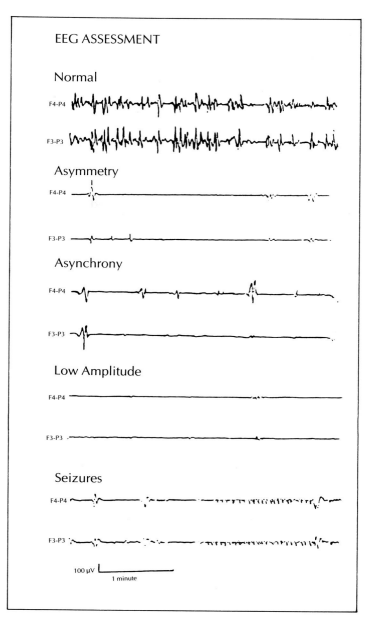

EEG ASSESSMENT

Normal

F4-P4

F3-P3

Asymmetry

F4-P4

F3-P3

Asynchrony

F4-P4

F3-P3

Low Amplitude

F4-P4

F3-P3

Seizures

F4-P4

F3-P3

100 μV

1 minute

The degree of maturation in any infant's tracing can then be related to these normal values. Other abnormalities in the EEG, such as seizure activity, excessively low voltage tracings, asymmetry and asynchrony, can also be detected (36). Sequential EEG recordings in infants with haemorrhagic and ischaemic lesions in the newborn period have shown that EEG changes may actually precede their appearance on ultrasound. The EEG is also a good prognostic indicator for a normal and abnormal outcome.

Doppler Ultrasound

The use of pulsed Doppler is well established in cardiological and obstetrical practice, and in recent years it has been used in the assessment of the cerebral circulation of both adults and newborn infants. Using a combined system with two dimensional imaging and pulsed Doppler ultrasound, individual vessels can be insonated repeatedly and changes in blood flow velocity determined. This approach is a potentially powerful tool in determining the pattern of cerebral blood flow associated with the development of haemorrhagic and ischaemic brain lesion in the newborn brain. As an example, **37** shows how blood velocity patterns alter in response to alterations in arterial carbon dioxide levels.

The technique is still being assessed and its place in the routine management of the sick newborn infant has not been established. It is, however, clearly important, when interpreting measurements of blood velocity in terms of blood flow, to have simultaneous information on heart rate, blood pressure and blood gases.

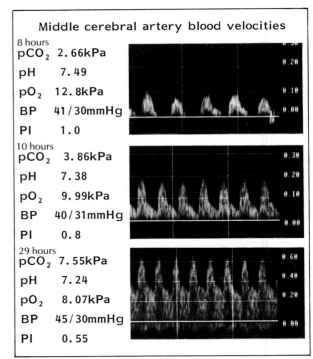

Middle cerebral artery blood velocities

8 hours	
pCO_2	2.66kPa
pH	7.49
pO_2	12.8kPa
BP	41/30mmHg
PI	1.0

10 hours	
pCO_2	3.86kPa
pH	7.38
pO_2	9.99kPa
BP	40/31mmHg
PI	0.8

29 hours	
pCO_2	7.55kPa
pH	7.24
pO_2	8.07kPa
BP	45/30mmHg
PI	0.55

Magnetic Resonance Imaging

Although a relatively new imaging technique, magnetic resonance imaging (MRI) is now recognised around the world as the diagnostic method of choice for examining the central nervous system. The lack of biological hazard, and the sensitivity to physiological and pathological change, make MRI an ideal method for the investigation of neonates and children.

We have used MRI to examine infants since 1982 and have had the opportunity to look at the normal development of the brain, including the progression of myelination and the early and late appearance of haemorrhagic and ischaemic lesions. MRI has been extremely useful in neonatal conditions, in helping to establish their timing and showing the late sequelae of the lesions after the closure of the anterior fontanelle, when ultrasound is no longer feasible. It can also be used to demonstrate the effect of the lesions on myelination.

The underlying physical principles for producing magnetic resonance images are given in Chapter 1, together with examples of the normal appearance of the developing brain with the techniques used in our hospital.

In the following chapters we aim to demonstrate that the combined use of all the different techniques provides a much more sensitive and comprehensive understanding than any individual method alone.

Chapter 1. Principles of Magnetic Resonance Imaging

A Glossary, References, and suggestions for Further Reading, referring to this Chapter, appear on page 194.

The Magnetic Resonance Phenomenon

When the nuclei of certain atoms are placed in a magnetic field they behave like tiny spinning bar magnets. The nuclei that do this are characterised by the fact that they have an odd number of protons or neutrons, and those of most medical interest are ^1H (protons), ^{23}Na, ^{31}P, ^{13}C and ^{19}F. Of these nuclei, protons are by far the most abundant and these have been of principal interest in magnetic resonance imaging (MRI).

When placed in an external *static magnetic field* the proton magnetisation aligns with the external magnetic field in much the same way as a compass needle does. This nuclear magnetisation differs from the compass needle because the protons' magnetisation is rotating; this is equivalent to the compass needle aligned in the field rotating about its long axis. The rate of rotation is directly proportional to the strength of the external field. For example, protons in the earth's magnetic field of 0.00005 *tesla* (T) rotate at the rate of about 2 kHz, whereas for imaging at 0.15 *tesla* the rate is 6.5 MHz.

If an additional magnetic field is applied perpendicular to the main magnetic field, then the direction of the nuclear magnetisation can be changed. This is similar to the way a compass needle can be deviated when another magnet is brought close to it. For the nuclear magnetisation this additional magnetic field must be applied at the rotational frequency of the nucleus. It is usual to create the magnetic field by using electrical currents with a frequency at the rate of the rotation of nuclei, i.e. 6.5 MHz (which is in the radiofrequency range) at 0.15 *tesla*. When this additional rotating magnetic field is applied the nuclear magnetisation (like a compass needle) can be tipped through any angle (**1**). It is most usual to rotate the magnetisation through 90° or through 180° (an inversion). When the rotating magnetic field is turned off the nuclear magnetisation returns to its equilibrium position. This return is described by two time constants T_1 and T_2. T_1 describes recovery in the direction of the large external static magnetic field and is known as longitudinal relaxation or spin lattice relaxation. T_2 describes recovery perpendicular to the main magnetic field and is known as transverse relaxation or spin spin relaxation. Both T_1 and T_2 depend on the local nuclear and molecular environment of the nuclei and thus on the chemical composition of the tissue or fluid. In the range of principal clinical interest, T_1 and T_2 are long for fluids (1,500–3,000 ms) but shorter for tissues (200–1,200 ms).

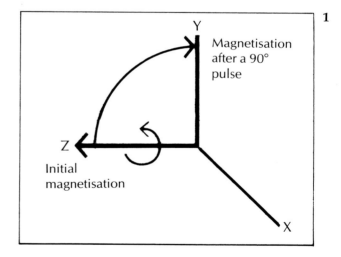

1

Y — Magnetisation after a 90° pulse

Z — Initial magnetisation

X

While the nuclear magnetisation is recovering back to its original position it represents a changing magnetic field and will induce a small current in a coil which is placed close to the nucleus. The current can then be amplified. This signal is known as the *Free induction decay*.

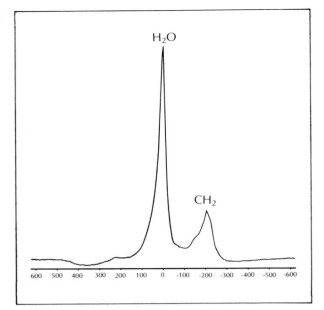

The rate of spinning of the nuclear magnetisation is slightly changed by the presence of electrons and other nuclei in the atomic or molecular locality. This is known as chemical shift. The frequencies are usually only changed by a few parts per million, but when displayed as a spectrum the shifts are often quite characteristic, and allow different chemical species to be identified (2*).

All matter is diamagnetic, paramagnetic or ferromagnetic. This means that, when placed in a magnetic field, all matter either slightly decreases the field (diamagnetic), slightly increases it (paramagnetic) or greatly increases it (ferromagnetic), relative to the magnetic field in a vacuum. The general term for this property is *magnetic susceptibility*. Most tissues of the body are diamagnetic, but some, including the breakdown products of haemoglobin, are paramagnetic. Tissues thus slightly decrease or increase the magnetic field when they are placed in it and this changes the spin frequency of the nuclear magnetisation.

If the magnetisations of several nuclei are spinning together in synchrony (i.e. they are in phase)

their magnetisations add together, whereas if they have slightly different spin frequencies (i.e. they are out of phase) their magnetisations tend to cancel out, leading to a net loss of detectable magnetisation.

If nuclei flow to a different magnetic field (and hence a different spin frequency) at different rates, then they become out of phase and there is usually a net loss of detectable voltage or signal in the surrounding coil.

To exploit these phenomena for imaging it is necessary to have a large static magnetic field, an additional rotating radiofrequency field to produce 90° and 180° pulses, gradient magnetic fields which can produce linear changes in magnetic field strength, and receiver coils. These requirements are dealt with in more detail in the next section.

Magnetic Resonance Imaging Equipment

Figure 3 illustrates a magnetic resonance imaging system. It is constructed around a large cylindrical *cryomagnet* (a) which produces a highly uniform magnetic field in the horizontal direction (the z axis). It is this magnetic field which aligns the magnetisation of the protons within the patient's body. At equilibrium this proton magnetisation points along the z axis.

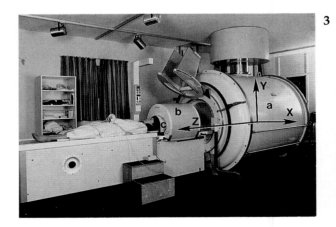

---

* Fig. 2 is a proton spectrum of the limb, displaying the water and fat peak.

In order to rotate this magnetisation through 90° or 180° an additional *transmitter coil* (b) is used. (The transmitter coil is usually fixed at the centre of the magnet.) This is turned on for short periods of time (typically about 1–2 ms) to rotate the proton magnetisation through 90° or 180° into the xy plane or the z direction.

As the magnetisation returns to its equilibrium position it induces a small current in the surrounding *receiver coil* (c).

An additional set of three orthogonal coils is necessary to encode spatially the current received from the nuclei. This is done by applying linear *gradient magnetic fields*. These magnetic fields uniformly increase in each of the x and y directions (for transverse images). This means that each nucleus is placed in a slightly different magnetic field and hence has a slightly different spin frequency; by identifying its spin frequency in the detected signal it is possible to determine where the nucleus is in space. This is a very fundamental principle. In fact it was this principle which made magnetic resonance imaging possible. To locate the nuclei in two dimensions, two sets of perpendicular magnetic fields are used.

The one remaining procedure necessary for imaging is a mechanism for selecting a slice. This is performed by applying a linear gradient magnetic field in the z direction, which produces a range of spin frequencies in the proton nuclei. The tipping magnetic field is then applied over a very limited range of spin frequencies, so only a limited range of nuclei respond or resonate. It is thus possible to select a narrow plane of responding protons and leave the other protons unaffected.

In imaging, the static field produces the net magnetisation, the rotating field changes its direction, the x and y gradient fields encode the information in space, and the z gradient coupled with a narrow range of spin frequencies selects the slice. The receiver coil detects the resultant voltage during the recovery or relaxation phase.

There is still considerable computer processing to be done using Fourier transformation, and the image must be displayed and archived. Overall control of the system is achieved by computer, and relatively simple instructions can be used to control these complex processes.

Properties of Magnetic Resonance Images: the Tissues

Unlike unenhanced X-ray computed tomography (CT) images which depend on a single parameter, the linear X-ray attenuation coefficient (μ), unenhanced magnetic resonance images depend on at least ten different physical properties. The most important of these are *proton density* (ρ), which is the number of protons per unit volume, T_1 and T_2, chemical shift, flow and susceptibility. We can analyse all the tissues of the human body in terms

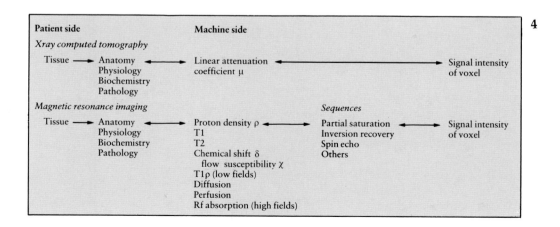

of these physical parameters and consider how a pathological change affects them. We can then relate the change in each parameter to the change in image signal intensity on the image via the pulse sequence. In the first stage we are looking at the 'patient' side of **4** and in the next section the 'machine' side. We will consider each of the first six parameters listed in **4** in turn.

Proton density actually refers to the mobile proton density, because protons must be in liquid or semi-liquid form to give an electrical signal. Water, cerebrospinal fluid (CSF) and urine have a proton density of 1, soft tissues 0.7–0.9, cartilage 0.2, cortical bone 0, and air 0. In many diseases proton density is increased: e.g. oedema. In other conditions, such as some types of fibrosis, proton density is decreased. The changes in proton density are usually of the order of 2–10%.

T_1 and T_2 reflect the viscosity of tissues, with pure water having a high value of T_1 and T_2 and soft tissues having a lower value. As the water content of a tissue increases, its T_1 and T_2 increase. This is the common change in disease. Another important determinant of T_1 and T_2 is the presence or absence of paramagnetic species. These decrease T_1 and T_2, so paramagnetic blood breakdown products typically have reduced values of T_1 and T_2.

Chemical shift effects are mostly of importance when considering protons in water, and protons in fat (triglycerides). The spin frequency of the two differs by 3.5 cycles per million. If the operating frequency is 6.5 MHz it is easy to calculate that it takes 22 ms for the signal from protons in water to become 180° out of phase with the signal from protons in fat. This is like two notes of music that are slightly out of tune. They 'beat' and, at a certain time, get out of phase with one another and cancel out. This cancellation effect is seen as dark lines at the boundary between water and fat on certain MR images.

Flow effects depend on the rate of flow, the type (laminar or turbulent), the direction, the phase of cardiac cycle and other factors. They are important in blood and CSF flow, joints, cysts and other fluid containing cavities.

Susceptibility effects are seen with paramagnetic species as mentioned before. They are also seen at interfaces between air and soft tissue or bone.

In the next section we outline how changes in these image parameters produce a change in image signal intensity by considering magnetic resonance pulse sequences.

Properties of Magnetic Resonance Images: the Pulse Sequences

The pulse sequences which we will discuss consist of a single 90° pulse (*Partial Saturation*, PS), a 90° pulse followed by a 180° pulse (*Spin Echo*, SE), and a 180° pulse followed by a 90° pulse (*Inversion Recovery*, IR).

With all three types of image the signal intensity is proportional to proton density. Thus the maxillary sinuses which contain air of zero proton density have zero signal with all three pulse sequences. Increases in proton density increase signal intensity (i.e. the tissue appears brighter), while reductions in proton density decrease signal intensity (i.e. the tissue appears darker).

The partial saturation sequence is used in T_1 and T_2 dependent forms. The T_2 dependence and the sensitivity to susceptibility effects are increased by increasing the echo time (*time to echo*, TE). This is the time from the 90° pulse to the point when the electrical signal is collected from the receiver coil (data collection). With TE values of 10 ms there is little T_2 dependence, but with values of 200 ms there is very strong T_2 dependence. Forms of the PS sequence of this type are used for detecting haemorrhage where the susceptibility effects lead to dephasing, producing a dark area due to loss of the signal.

Spin echo sequences are mainly dependent on T_1 or T_2. They are most often used in the T_2 dependent form to detect the increase in T_2 seen in a wide variety of diseases. These regions appear as bright areas on T_2 dependent images.

Inversion recovery images are used in two main forms. The first is the medium TI form (*inversion time*, the time from the 180° pulse to the 90°) with T_1 about 500–800 ms. This is highly T_1 dependent. Tissues having an increase in T_1 appear dark with this sequence in contradistinction to the T_2 spin echo sequence, where the increase in T_2 makes such lesions appear light. The second form of the inversion recovery sequence has a short TI (100 ms), and this behaves more like a spin echo sequence, with tissues with an increase in T_1 or T_2 appearing light.

The notation for these sequences follows the American College of Radiology recommendations.

Patient Preparation and Safety

We examine neonates and infants of less than three months after a feed and during natural sleep. Children aged from three months to two years are given oral chloral hydrate (80–100 mg/kg) via a naso–gastric tube, thus ensuring that a known amount of sedative is received. Children from three to four years are given the same dose of oral chloral hydrate in fruit juice. Older children are not sedated but are given a call button to press if they want to talk to the staff during the scan.[1] If they are very anxious, a member of staff accompanies them inside the magnet. Most children over five years find a magnetic resonance scan an acceptable procedure and lie still for its duration.

The magnet is a large piece of equipment relative to the size of a tiny baby, and parents may appear a little apprehensive at letting their infants enter the 'giant tunnel'. The National Radiological Protection Board (NRPB) has provided guidelines for the use of magnetic resonance in clinical practice.[2] To date, magnetic resonance is believed to be without biological hazard if operated within these guidelines, so parents are encouraged to be present while the child is prepared, positioned and examined.

A surface respiratory monitor is attached to the abdomen of sedated infants so that breathing patterns can be observed from outside the magnet. In rare instances a general anaesthetic is used; this is not a hazardous procedure from a magnetic resonance point of view if metal-free intubation equipment is used and the equipment is kept at a safe distance from the magnet.

The infants are swaddled for warmth and security and their heads are placed in a closely fitting receiver coil in the shape of a space helmet (5). These coils are available in a variety of sizes to accommodate the increasing head size of the growing child (6).

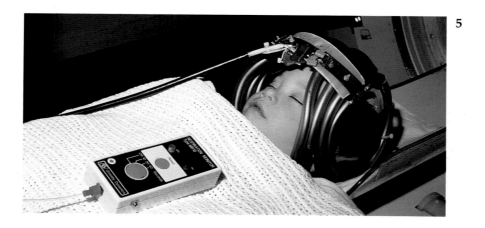

5

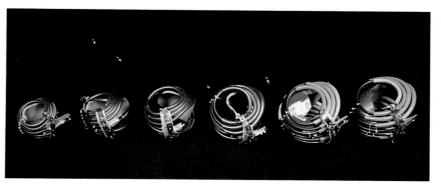

6

Most children are examined supine; however, if there is the slightest risk of inhalation of vomit or mucous, they are placed laterally.

Possible hazards considered by the NRPB include heating of tissues by the radiofrequency fields, induced currents in the body from the changing magnetic field gradients and the static field *per se*. Loose metal objects may be attracted to the magnet and hit the patient. All loose metal objects must therefore be removed from patients and accompanying persons. Babies are always checked twice for nappy pins and metal poppers.

Normal Appearances of the Brain

At birth the infant brain contains 95% water and it has a very long T_1 and T_2 relaxation time. There is a rapid fall in water content to 82–84% during the first two years of life, as physiological myelination takes place. The corresponding fall in T_1 values in a series of normal infants plotted against age is shown in **7**.

It is necessary to adjust the timing of the pulse sequences accordingly. For example, in the neonatal period a *TR* of 3000 ms and *TI* of 1000 ms are required to produce an inversion recovery scan with useful soft tissue contrast.

The *TR* and *TI* can be halved by the time the child is two years of age, as the water content of the brain approaches that of an adult. The parameters of the sequences used for imaging children in a 0.15 *tesla* system are given below.

Sequence	TR	TI	TE
Partial saturation	1500		33
	1660		113
	1660		193
spin echo (T_1 dependent)	544		44
(T_2 dependent)	1500		120
Inversion recovery			
<40 weeks	3000	1000	44
0–2 months	2400	800	44
3 months–2 years	1800	600	44
2 years and over	1500	500	44
short TI inversion recovery	1500	100	44

The process of myelination begins *in utero* and is visible with the naked eye at 32 weeks in the posterior limb of the internal capsule. It progresses rapidly during the first two years of life and continues slowly well into the second decade. Myelination has been well documented in pathological specimens by Yakovlev and Lecours in 1967[3] (**8**), but magnetic resonance offers the opportunity to study this process during life.

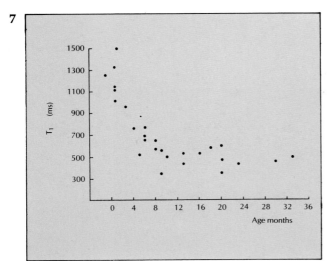

7

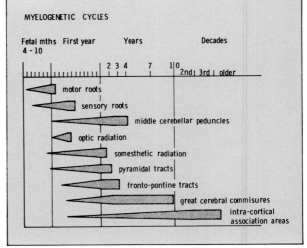

8

Progressive myelination is well shown with inversion recovery sequences. 9–12 are sequential scans in a normal term infant. These low resolution images were produced in 1982 before any technical developments to improve image quality were implemented. At two weeks of age myelin is visible in the thalamus, and areas of low signal intensity (dark) are seen in the periventricular regions (arrows). Little structure is seen in the brain parenchyma with these low resolution images (9).

At an age of two and a half months the areas of long T_1 are less prominent and a little more myelin is seen (10).

At six months myelin is apparent in the internal and external capsule as well as posteriorly in the occipito-thalamic radiation (11). By 10 months a further increase in white matter has occurred anteriorly and posteriorly (12), and the forceps major and minor are myelinated.

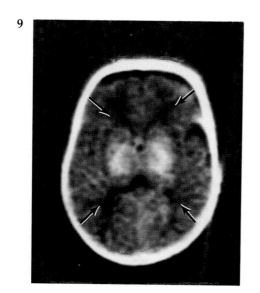

9

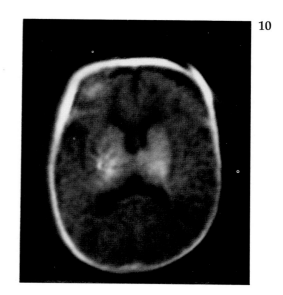

10

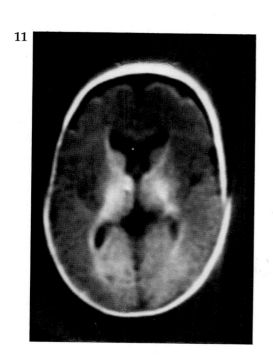

11

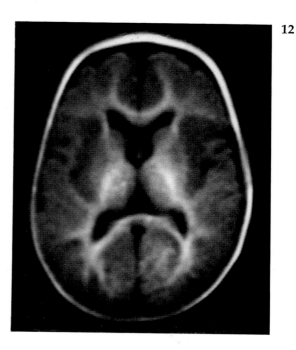

12

In the neonatal period, unmyelinated white matter has a lower signal intensity than grey matter, and the cortical mantle appears highlighted against the cerebrospinal fluid outside the brain (13) with inversion recovery sequences. Between six and 12 months the T_1 of unmyelinated white matter becomes equal to that of grey matter. As more myelin is laid down, the signal intensity from white matter becomes greater than that from grey matter (14).

The advantages of higher spatial resolution imaging are obvious; however, caution must be exercised when comparisons are made between images done with different techniques. For example, in 12 and 15 both infants are 10 months old, and the level of myelination is probably not sig-

nificantly different, but all structures within the brain are more clearly defined in 15 – which is the high resolution image.

By three years of age, further myelination has taken place, especially anteriorly and laterally, with higher signal intensity anteriorly rather than posteriorly (16).

At nine years, myelination is almost complete (17). The adult brain is shown in 18. The temporalis muscle (moderate signal intensity) has developed, and high signal intensity can be seen from bone marrow in the diploic space.

A black or white dot with shadowing through the central axis is present on some images – this is an artefact due to the reconstruction process. Movement artefacts appear as alternating dark

13

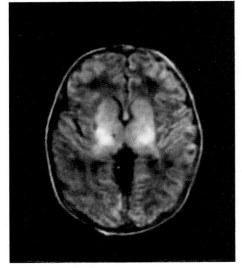

14

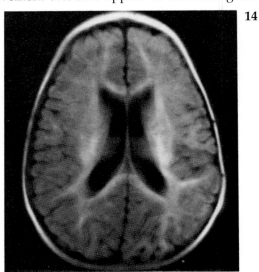

15

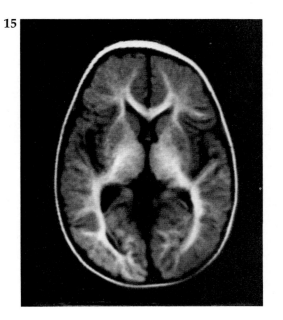

16

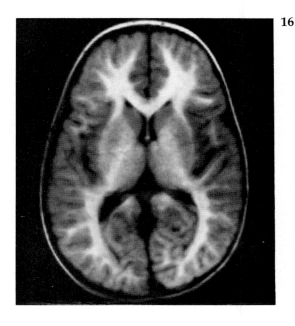

and light bands across the background. Ventriculo–peritoneal shunts produce a U-shaped artefact.

There is also a loss in signal intensity in the immediate vicinity of a shunt tract.

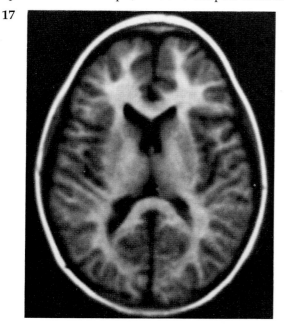

17

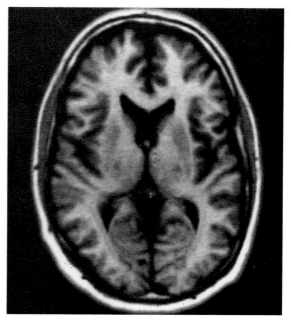

18

Pathological Appearances of the Brain

The theoretical basis for changes in magnetic resonance images in disease was outlined above. In this section, some of the changes seen in disease are illustrated. Knowledge of pathological change in diseases of children is rapidly increasing.[4, 5]

In **19**, a partial saturation sequence displays grey/white matter contrast, with grey matter of lower signal intensity than white matter. Cerebrospinal fluid signal is greater than brain, a result of the very much longer T_2 of CSF. In the case illustrated an intracerebral haemorrhage is shown as a high signal intensity area on the inversion recovery image (**20**), and an area of changed susceptibility appears in **21**. The black and white alternating bands in this image and all susceptibility maps used in this atlas are due to inhomogeneities in the main external static field.

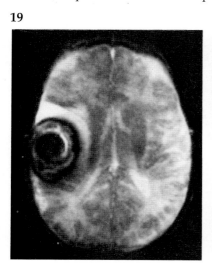

19

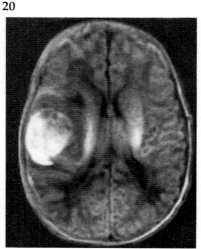

20

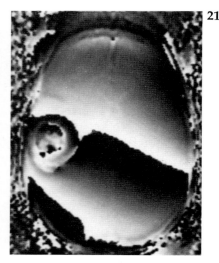

21

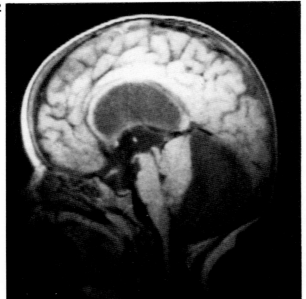

22

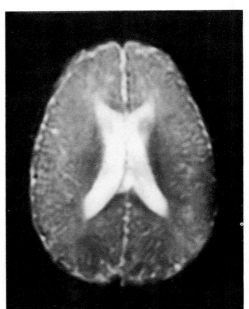

23

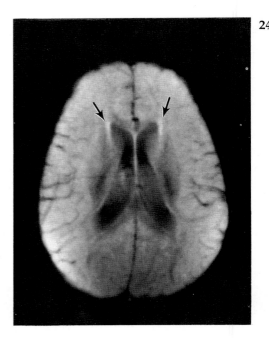

24

Spin echo images can be weighted to display either T_1 or T_2 dependent effects. The T_1 dependent image displays relatively little soft tissue contrast, with the signal from CSF less than that from brain. It is useful to show anatomical detail such as the cerebellar cyst in this child with Dandy Walker syndrome (22). The T_2 weighted spin echo sequence tends to show a CSF signal equal to that of brain or greater (23). Pathological features are usually shown as increased signal intensity, and there may be difficulty in identifying periventricular lesions when the CSF signal is greater than that of brain.

The short TI inversion recovery sequence suppresses the signal from fat containing tissues and the contrast of the remaining tissues depends on the sum of the T_1 and T_2 effects. The cerebrospinal fluid has moderate signal intensity and contrasts well with the low signal intensity of the white matter. Grey matter is displayed with moderate to high signal intensity. Vascular structures are seen with low signal intensity. Pathology is generally highlighted (arrows) (24).

The medium TI inversion recovery sequence shows a high level of grey/white matter contrast. Cerebrospinal fluid is displayed as low signal intensity (dark). Grey matter appears as moderate signal (grey), and white matter and subcutaneous fat have high signal intensity (bright). Inversion recovery images have been most useful for following the developmental pattern of myelination (e.g. 15–18) and delays of deficits in this process. Pathology generally appears dark with this sequence.

Chapter 2. Intraventricular and Periventricular Haemorrhage

Historical Background

Ruckenstein and Zollner (1929) were the first to recognise that in premature infants blood in the ventricles occurred as the result of a haemorrhage in the germinal matrix.

Pathological Features

In the premature infant, 90% of haemorrhages occur into the germinal matrix at the head of the caudate nucleus, adjacent to the foramen of Monro. In 50%, the lesion is bilateral, but left sided lesions may be slightly more common; blood will rupture into the lateral ventricle in a large number of cases, and involvement of the brain parenchyma may occur. The latter can be related to bleeding into an ischaemic area or to venous infarction. Posthaemorrhagic ventricular dilatation and the evolution of a parenchymal lesion into a porencephalic cyst can be seen when the infants survive for longer.

Clinical Recognition

Ultrasound is the method of choice for the diagnosis of these lesions. Haemorrhage can be recognised on ultrasound for several weeks. Sequential scans allow the recognition of posthaemorrhagic ventricular dilatation and a porencephalic cyst. Measurements of the ventricles can be taken at regular intervals to time appropriately the need for active intervention.

Figures **1–6** illustrate the grading of haemorrhages on ultrasound in coronal and parasagittal views. (i) Grade I haemorrhage is localised to the germinal layer (**1** and **4**). (ii) Grade II haemorrhage extends into the basal ganglia (**2** and **5**). Also there is usually blood in the lateral ventricles. A grade IIa haemorrhage exists when there is only a small amount of blood in the ventricular system: a grade IIb haemorrhage occurs when 50% or more of the ventricular system is filled with blood. (iii) In a grade III haemorrhage, there is blood in the ventricles which communicates with blood in the brain parenchyma (**3** and **6**).

1 2 3

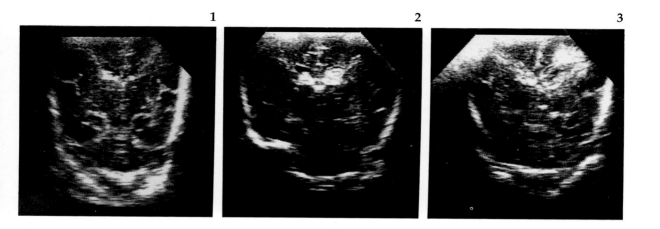

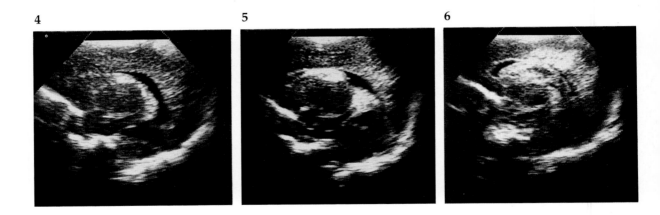

X-ray Computed Tomography: On CT, haemorrhage appears as an area of high attenuation for approximately one week after the initial bleed, then it may become isodense with the brain parenchyma and be difficult to recognise.

Magnetic Resonance Imaging: The appearance of haemorrhage with MRI varies with the pulse sequence and time of the examination from the initial bleed.

Clinical examination: Infants with intraventricular haemorrhages show a typical behavioural pattern in the acute and the recovery phase.

One of the common signs in the early stages of intraventricular haemorrhage is a relatively tight popliteal angle relative to leg tone elicited by traction. Figure **7** shows poor tone in the limb on traction but the popliteal angle is only 100° compared to the expected 150°–170° (**8**). The presence of this sign is independent of the size of the haemorrhage. It occurs within the first 48 hours or may even precede the recognition of the haemorrhage on ultrasound. It usually resolves within a week. During that time the infants are also very hypotonic. This is seen in supine posture (**9**), ventral suspension (**10**) and sitting (**11**). While limb hypotonia improves rapidly, trunk hypotonia persists for several weeks. Not only is general maturation of tone often delayed in these infants but there is also a delay in visual function.

The progression of clinical signs in infants with periventricular/intraventricular haemorrhage is tabulated, *right*.

Although these clinical signs are common in periventricular/intraventricular haemorrhage they appear to have no prognostic significance.

Asymmetry of tone may also be present in those infants who develop a large porencephalic cyst, which is an early indication of hemiplegia.

Haemorrhage: Progression of Clinical Signs

Stage I

- no auditory response
- arm recoil > leg recoil
- excessive motility
- ± abnormal Moro
- tendon reflexes increased
- no orientation

Stage II

- ± auditory response
- decreased tone
- popliteal angle tight
- decreased motility
- no tremor or startle
- no visual orientation
- poor reactivity

Stage III

- auditory response normal
- limb tone normal
- popliteal angle normal
- decreased head control
- decreased motility
- ± visual orientation
- ± roving eye movements

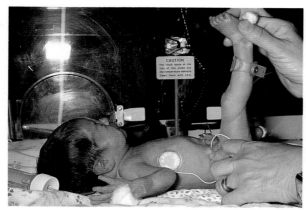

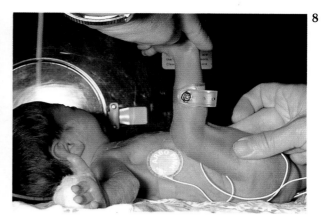

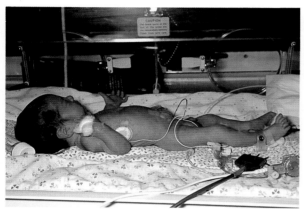

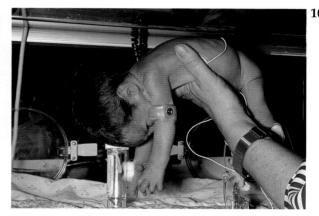

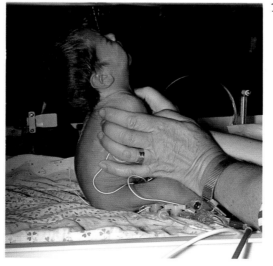

Electrophysiological Tests

Auditory Brainstem Evoked Responses (ABR):
In the first week following the onset of the haemorrhage the brainstem evoked response is usually abnormal and often absent. Recovery generally occurs over the next 2–4 weeks, despite the presence of concomitant posthaemorrhagic ventricular dilation.

Visual Evoked Responses (VER): A delay in maturation is frequently present. An early positivity usually appears between 30 and 33 weeks postmenstrual age in normal premature infants. However, in premature infants with haemorrhages, the positivity is often delayed to 36–40 weeks postmenstrual age. Figure **12** compares the VER of a normal premature infant with that of an infant with intraventricular haemorrhage at a comparable postmenstrual age. The findings in the neonatal period are usually symmetrical, even in the presence of large unilateral lesions. Asymmetry is more common after 48–52 weeks postmenstrual age.

Somatosensory Evoked Response (SER): A delay in latency of the negative wave is frequently present, as shown in **13**. In progressive ventricular dilation, there is a decrease in latency and an increase in amplitude after the insertion of a shunt.

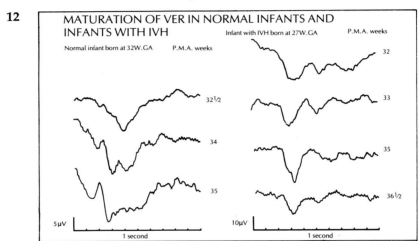

12

MATURATION OF VER IN NORMAL INFANTS AND INFANTS WITH IVH

Normal infant born at 32W.GA   P.M.A. weeks

Infant with IVH born at 27W.GA   P.M.A. weeks

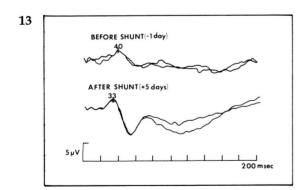

13

BEFORE SHUNT(-1day)
40

AFTER SHUNT(+5 days)
33

5 μV

200 msec

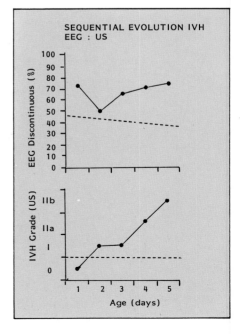

14

SEQUENTIAL EVOLUTION IVH
EEG : US

Electroencephalogram (EEG): Early continuous EEG recording may demonstrate abnormalities of cerebral function preceding the ultrasound evolution of the haemorrhage or the extension of the haemorrhage (**14**). It also provides a sensitive guide to prognosis and can be particularly valuable in lesions where ultrasound is of indeterminate predictive value.

Case Histories

The following case histories illustrate the value of the above techniques in three children who died, and in nine premature infants and two term infants who survived, with periventricular and/or intraventricular haemorrhage.

Case 1

Premature infant, born at 29 weeks gestation, who weighed 680 grams at birth (<3rd centile). She required ventilation for severe hyaline membrane disease. A large intraventricular haemorrhage was diagnosed on day 3 shortly before she died.

The **ultrasound** examinations were normal during the first three days, but a scan before death showed bilateral intraventricular haemorrhage with probable parenchymal extension on the right (**15**).

A **CT** scan was done after the child had died. There were high attenuation regions in the lateral ventricles and a suggestion of haemorrhage spreading into the brain parenchyma from the right anterior horn of the ventricle (**16**).

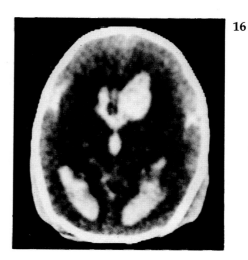

16

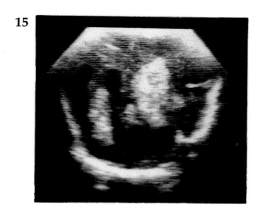

15

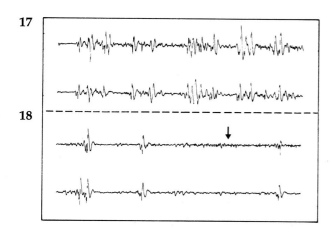

17

18

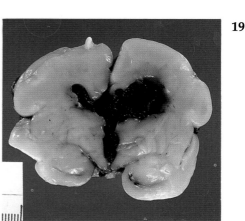

19

Electroencephalogram: Continuous 4-channel EEG done on day 1 when the ultrasound was normal showed excessive discontinuity over 24 hours (**17**). On the second day, excessive discontinuity was seen on the right (**18**), preceding the extension of the haemorrhage by 24 hours.

Macroscopic examination showed dilatation of the right anterior horn of the ventricle, but no haemorrhage in the brain parenchyma (**19**).

Comment: Germinal layer haemorrhages often rupture into the ventricles to produce intraventricular haemorrhage, and the brain parenchyma may also be involved. This case illustrates that it can be difficult to be certain about parenchymal involvement, which was suspected on ultrasound and CT in this case but was not seen on the post-mortem specimen.

Case 2

The **ultrasound** scan of a premature infant, born at 27 weeks gestation, showed bilateral parenchymal involvement (**20**).

Periventricular areas of increased echogenicity were seen separate from the ventricles before the parenchymal spread occurred.

At autopsy the meninges were congested, with a yellowish tinge. There was a subarachnoid clot in the cisterna magna and over the lower surface of the cerebellum, with spread over the base of the brain and into the Sylvian fissure. Coronal sections of the cerebrum showed massive bilateral intraventricular haemorrhage arising from subependymal haemorrhage, with extensive involvement of the parenchyma on the left (**21**).

Comment: Even when there is no doubt that the brain parenchyma is involved, it is not always possible to be certain about the underlying mechanism of the haemorrhage on the basis of ultrasound alone. In this case the parenchymal haemorrhage presumably occurred in the previously ischaemic areas.

20

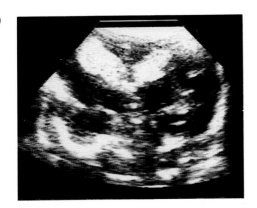

21

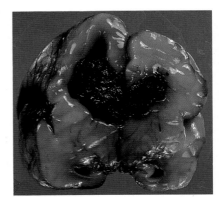

Case 3

This infant, born at 27 weeks gestation, showed involvement of the brain parenchyma which was different in shape from case 2 (**22**).

At autopsy the coronal section of the cerebrum showed a large subependymal and moderate intraventricular haemorrhage on the right. The haemorrhage was associated with intense venous congestion in the periventricular white matter (**23**). Note the dilated veins at the upper right hand margin of the haemorrhage.

Comment: The extension of the haemorrhage in this case was due to venous infarction.

22

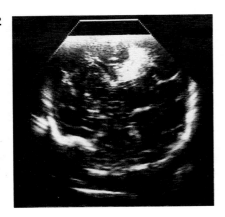

23

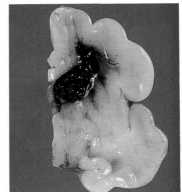

Case 4

Premature infant, second of twins born by vaginal breech delivery at 30 weeks gestation. He was asphyxiated at birth and had severe respiratory distress syndrome. He developed large bilateral intraventricular haemorrhage with post haemorrhagic ventricular dilatation. He was normal at follow up at 18 months of age.

Ultrasound: The first scan at 10 hours of age was unremarkable. At 20 hours, after an acute clinical deterioration, more than 50% of the lateral ventricles were filled by large casts (**24** and **25**). No involvement of the brain parenchyma was seen.

24

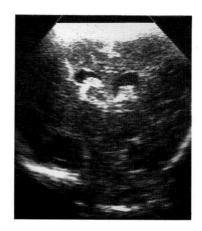

25

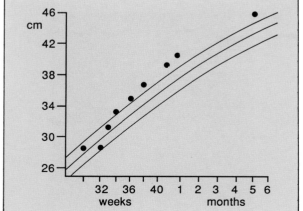

26

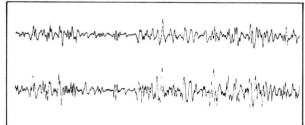

Electroencephalogram: At the time the haemorrhage occurred a continuous 4-channel EEG recording (**26**) was normal and remained normal.

He developed further posthaemorrhagic ventricular dilatation (**27**). Lumbar taps were not performed on a regular basis, but two lumbar punctures were carried out because of an excessive increase in head circumference (**28**).

27

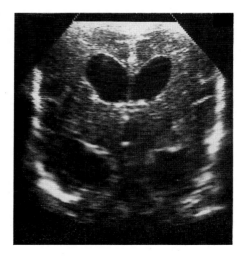

28

There was no further increase in the size of the ventricles after three weeks of age, but persistent ventricular dilatation was still noted on his ultrasound scan at one year (29).

Clinical examination: At 40 weeks postmenstrual age the infant was hypotonic in the supine position (30), when pulled to sit (31) and in ventral suspension (32). Note also the degree of head lag in 31 and the unusual degree of flexion of the arms for an infant of 40 weeks postmenstrual age. However, over-abducted posture of the hips is normal in premature infants at this age (31). When held in a sitting position, an increase in neck extensor tone was also noted (33). His Moro response was immature, consisting mainly of full abduction (34).

29

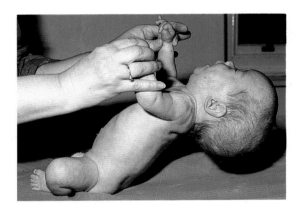

31

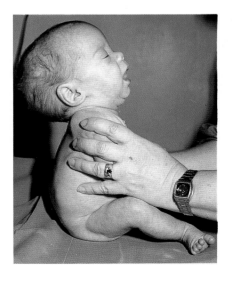

33

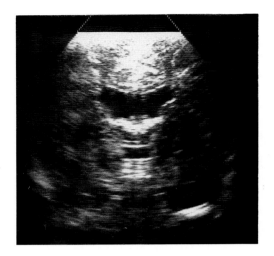

30

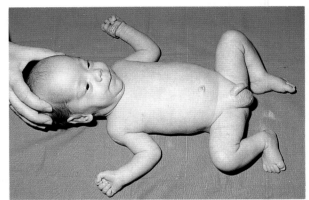

32

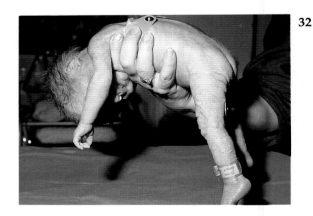

34

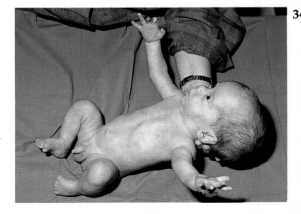

At seven months he was active, played with his toes (35), but was still hypotonic when held standing (36), and exhibited poor trunk control when held in a sitting position (37). At 18 months he was able to walk unaided (38).

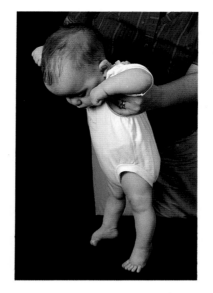

36

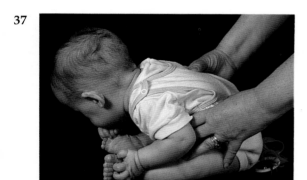

35

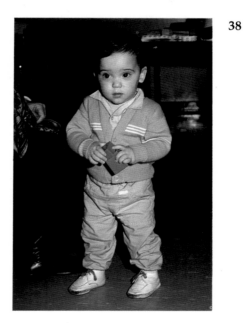

38

37

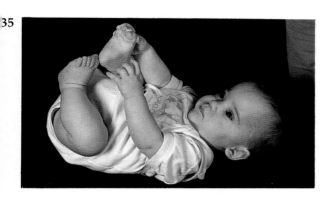

Comment: This case illustrates that ultrasound can be very useful to monitor the increase in ventricular dilatation. Measurements of the ventricles can be made as long as the fontanelle remains open. This child had a normal 4-channel EEG despite being critically ill. These early normal findings appear to correlate well with a normal outcome. On clinical examination, children with intraventricular haemorrhages often remain hypotonic for prolonged periods, but this is not prognostic, and they tend to normalise despite the initial developmental delay.

All ages at follow up clinical examination are given as chronological age uncorrected for prematurity.

Case 5

Premature infant, second of twins (the first twin was stillborn), born at 32 weeks gestation by vaginal breech delivery. He was ventilated for the first three days for respiratory distress syndrome. He developed large bilateral intraventricular haemorrhages, with periventricular echogenicities, but he had a completely normal outcome at two years of age.

Ultrasound examination was normal on the first and second days of life. Large bilateral intra-ventricular haemorrhages were demonstrated on day 3. Marked echogenic areas in continuity with the ventricles were seen around the wall of the right lateral ventricle, in the coronal (39) and parasagittal views (arrows) (40). Mild ventricular dilatation occurred at two weeks and small cystic lesions were seen adjacent to the wall of the lateral ventricles (arrow) (41). After a short time the cysts were no longer visible, as presumably they disappeared into the dilated ventricles.

39

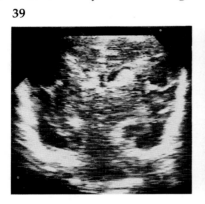

40

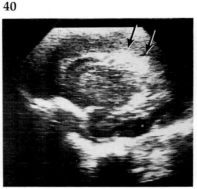

41

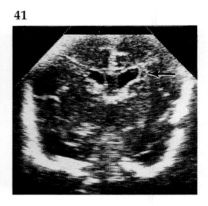

42

Auditory Brainstem Evoked Responses: On day 4 responses were present, but the waveshapes were poor, especially on the left, and the I–V interpeak latency was prolonged. On day 20 there was an improvement in wave shapes and a decrease in the latencies was seen despite the ventricular dilatation (42).

Visual Evoked Responses showed delayed maturation and a positivity was still absent at 39 weeks postmenstrual age (**43**).

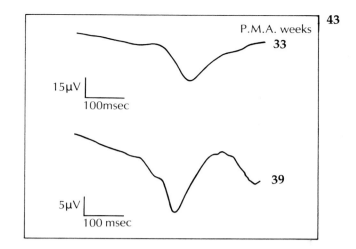

Clinical examination at 34 weeks postmenstrual age showed marked hypotonia. Severe head lag was present when the child was pulled to sit (**44**), and in ventral suspension (**45**). The tone in his limbs was markedly decreased for an infant of this postmenstrual age (**46**).

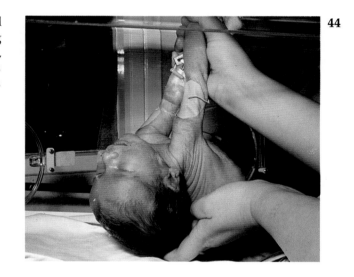

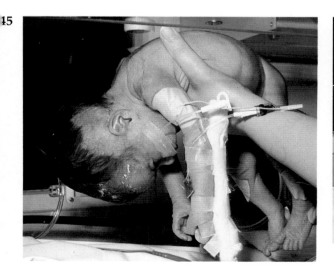

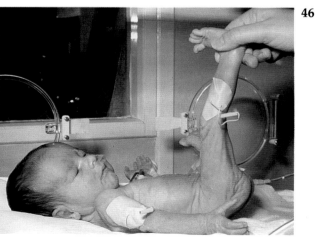

However, he sat at seven months (**47**), walked unaided at 13 months (**48**), and played stooping on the floor at 24 months (**49**).

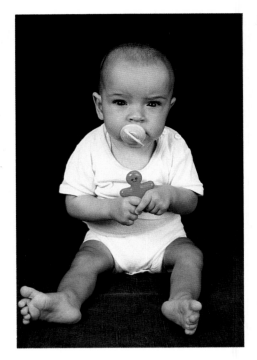

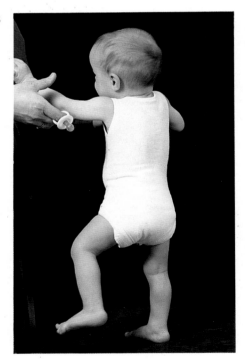

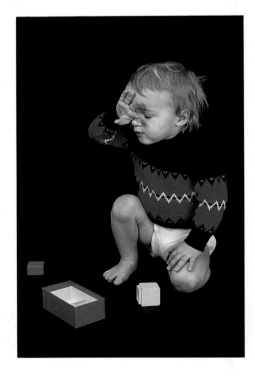

His head circumference crossed the 50th and the 90th centile between one and six months of age, although the ventricular dilatation was stable. The head circumference continued to grow above, but parallel to, the 90th centile (**50**).

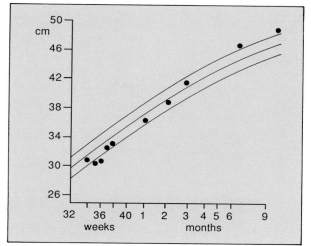

Magnetic Resonance Imaging: At 20 months myelination was within normal limits on the inversion recovery scan. The ventricles were also within normal limits except for a slight enlargement of the right occipital horn (**51**).

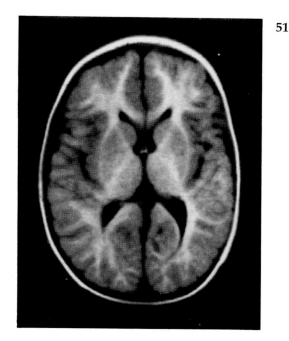

Comment: This case illustrates a number of important points: (i) the difficulty in classifying parenchymal densities and predicting their subsequent evolution; (ii) prolonged hypotonia is common in infants with intraventricular haemorrhage, but is not a marker for poor outcome; (iii) the delay in the maturation of the visually evoked potentials is a frequent finding in infants with IVH, but it is not necessarily related to the presence of occipital involvement, nor does it predict later visual or neurological abnormality.

Case 6

Premature infant, born at 28 weeks gestation by an elective caesarean section for *placenta praevia*. The child was 'flat' at birth with Apgar scores of 1 and 7 at one and five minutes respectively. He developed severe hyaline membrane disease and required ventilation for the first 16 days. His course was complicated by bilateral pneumothoraces. He developed bilateral intraventricular haemorrhages with a unilateral area of increased echogenicity on the right, but his clinical development was normal.

Ultrasound examinations were normal on day 1, but a bilateral intraventricular haemorrhage with casts was noted on day 2, as well as an area of increased echogenicity adjacent to the right ventricle (**52**) (arrow). Three weeks later, mild ventricular dilatation was present and the echogenic area had become cystic (**53**). The cysts were also clearly seen on the parasagittal view (**54**) (arrow).

52　　　　　　**53**　　　　　　**54**

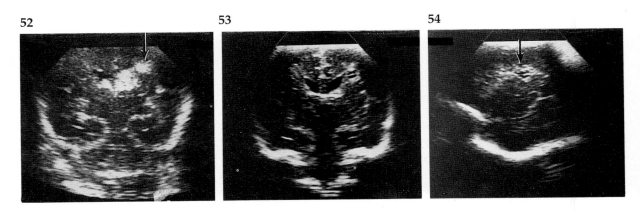

55

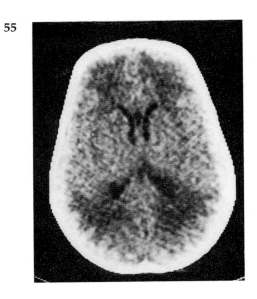

A **CT** scan at 35 weeks postmenstrual age showed areas of generalised decreased attenuation in the periventricular regions but no localised cystic lesions (**55**).

Clinical examination: At nine months he had normal development and he was able to crawl on hands and knees (**56**).

Magnetic Resonance Imaging: Inversion recovery sequences at 12 months of age are shown. Myelination was within normal limits and there was a slight asymmetry in ventricular shape (**57**). At the level of the centrum semiovale, an area of low signal intensity (dark) (arrows) was present on the right anteriorly (**58**).

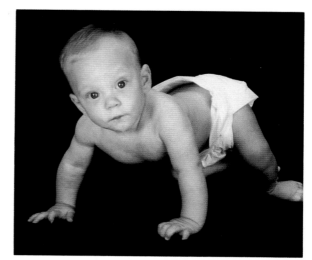

56

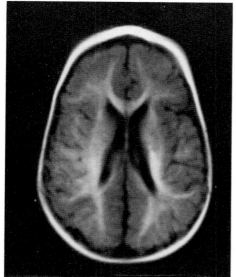

57

58

Comment: The lesion seen on ultrasound in the mid coronal view corresponds to a lesion in the parietal region in the parasagittal view (**54**). It is noteworthy that the cysts which were clearly seen on ultrasound were not apparent on the CT. This infant had no motor deficit despite the lesion in the centrum semiovale. Lesions in this area are thought to relate to later cerebral palsy. The normal development in this child may have been due to the unilateral involvement and the relatively small size of the lesion.

Case 7

Preterm infant, born at 26 weeks gestation following prolonged rupture of membranes, with evidence of amnionitis. An intraventricular haemorrhage with an area of periventricular echogenicity on the left was seen on the first ultrasound scan a few hours after delivery. At 12 months the infant showed only slight asymmetry and no other abnormality.

Ultrasound examination three hours after birth showed a marked intraventricular haemorrhage on the left and areas of increased echogenicity around the external angles of the lateral ventricles in the coronal view, with the scan head angled backwards (**59**) (arrow). The parasagittal view showed blood in the ventricle (**60**) but no evidence of parenchymal extension. No cysts developed and the ventricles did not increase in size.

Clinical examination: A slight asymmetry in tone was seen at 12 months. He preferred to use his left hand (**61**) and the popliteal angle on the right was slightly tighter than on the left (**62**).

59

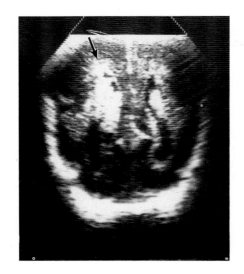

60

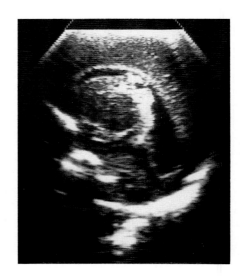

61

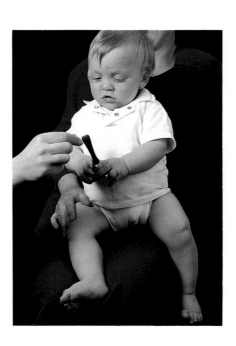

62

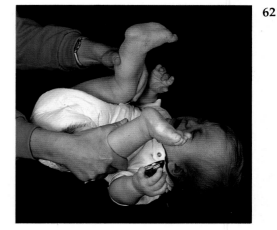

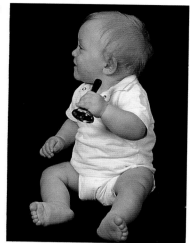

63

However, he was able to sit well and pivot (**63**), and crawl on hands and knees (**64**). He required only slight support to stand (**65**).

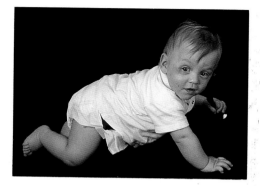

64

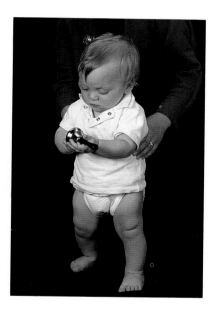

65

Comment: It is of interest that, although this infant showed periventricular densities similar to Cases 5 and 6, these densities did not evolve into cystic lesions. In contrast to Cases 5 and 6, this child later developed mild asymmetry in tone and movement. Permission for the MRI study was not obtained, and it is not known if the child's asymmetry of tone was due to a lesion other than the one seen with ultrasound.

Note also that this infant had a large lesion diagnosed on the first ultrasound performed within three hours of birth, a feature seen more frequently in infants when the mother has amnionitis.

Case 8

Premature infant, born at 28 weeks gestation. She required ventilation for the first 48 hours for apnoeic spells. She developed a large intraventricular haemorrhage with parenchymal involvement, which evolved into a porencephalic cyst. She was completely normal at two years of age.

Ultrasound examination was normal on day 1. The following day a large intraventricular haemorrhage was visible involving the brain parenchyma on the left (**66**). Three weeks later a porencephalic cyst developed at the site of the parenchymal haemorrhage (**67**).

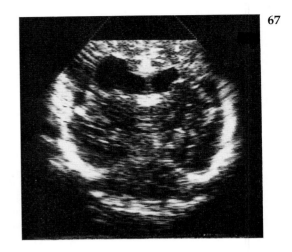

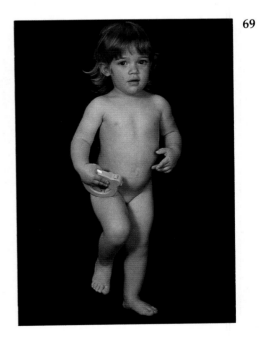

Clinical examination: At 13 months her development was appropriate for her age and no asymmetry in tone could be elicited. She was able to sit and pivoted well (**68**). At 18 months she walked unaided (**69**) and did not show any asymmetry in tone.

Magnetic Resonance Imaging: At three years of age the ventricles were mildly dilated and a small porencephalic cyst was seen anteriorly on the left on the inversion recovery sequence. Myelination was within normal limits but there was less myelin in the left hemisphere than in the right (**70**). The short TI inversion recovery sequence at the same level displayed the cyst but only minor periventricular changes (arrow) (**71**).

70

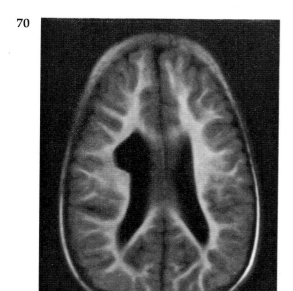

71

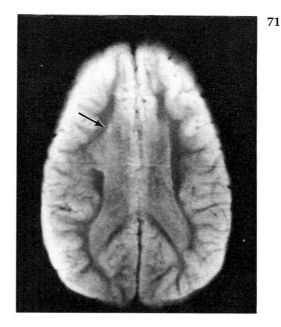

Comment: This case shows that infants with parenchymal lesions, which evolve into a porencephalic cyst, may show a delay or deficit in myelination on the side of the porencephalic cyst but be free from any abnormal neurological signs at follow up.

Case 9

Premature infant, first of twins, born at 29 weeks gestation. She had severe hyaline membrane disease and was ventilated for 14 days. She developed a large intraventricular haemorrhage with parenchymal involvement. On clinical examination at three years of age she had a hemiplegia and normal intellect.

Ultrasound: Her initial ultrasound scan was normal but a large intraventricular and parenchymal haemorrhage was seen on day 3. A large porencephalic cyst evolved during the next four weeks (**72**) with concomitant ventricular dilatation, seen in the coronal view with the scan head angled backwards (**73**).

She had repeated lumbar and ventricular taps, and a graph showing sequential head circumference measurements is shown in **74**, illustrating the effects of the taps.

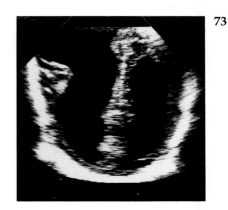

72   **73**

74

Head circumference and ventricular index

L = Lumbar puncture
V = Ventricular tap
OFC = Occipito-frontal circumference
VI = Ventricular index

Auditory Brainstem Evoked Responses at 36 weeks postmenstrual age were normal.

Visual Evoked Responses: at 35 weeks the responses were symmetrical, despite a unilateral lesion. At six and nine months an asymmetry was present (**75**).

Clinical examination at 37 weeks showed a marked degree of hypotonia, which was readily observed in the supine position (**76**). Compared with her twin sister (**77**) she showed poor neck flexion (**78**).

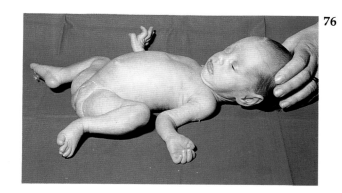

75

R   age 40 days

L

5µV

R   age 6 months

L

15µV

R   age 9 months

L

20µV
        1 second

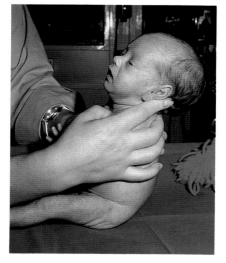

77

78

Differences between the twins at six months were also seen in ventral suspension (79 and 80). When the affected child had her legs extended, she was unable to elevate her head above the plane of her body (79). The normal twin showed flexed legs and she could hold her head above the plane of her body in the same position (80). At nine months the affected twin showed a marked asymmetry of her popliteal angles (81) and she preferred using her left hand (82), but she was able to grasp a ring with her right hand (83).

79
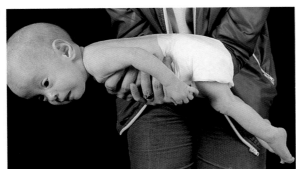

80
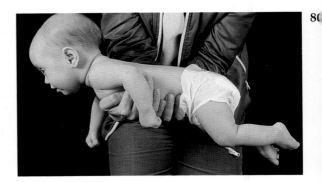

81
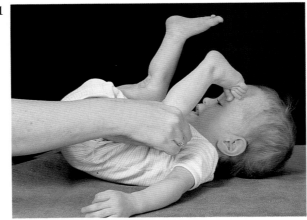

Aged 17 months she managed to take a few steps on her own; her sister was walking well at this stage (**84**). Mental development was very satisfactory in both girls. The affected child performed at an appropriate level for her age on the Griffiths developmental test (**85**), and during this test she used her right hand from time to time. Aged three she developed convulsions which were associated with febrile episodes. Subsequently she developed convulsions without fever for which she receives treatment.

82

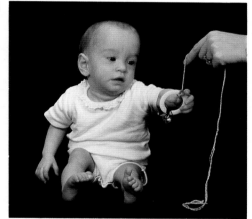

83

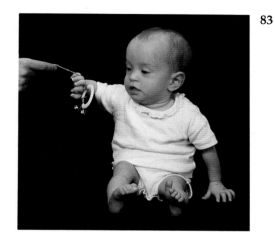

84

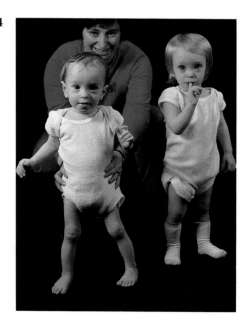

85

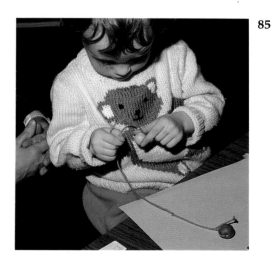

Magnetic Resonance Imaging: Inversion recovery sequences are shown in both infants at 12 and 36 months. In the unaffected child the ventricular system was normal and myelination was at the expected level for a 12-month-old infant (**86**). An increase in white matter was seen at three years (**87**).

The affected child at 12 months showed ventricular dilatation and a large left anterior porencephalic cyst. Less myelin was seen in the left hemisphere than in the right (**88**). Aged three years there was little change in the configuration or size of the ventricles; however, there had been a considerable increase in the level of white matter, especially on the right (**89**). Myelination was delayed compared with her sister on both occasions. The partial saturation sequence showed low signal intensity in the periventricular regions (arrows) on the right (**90**). The susceptibility map (**91**) showed phase changes at the sites of the low signal in **90**, indicative of previous haemorrhage.

86

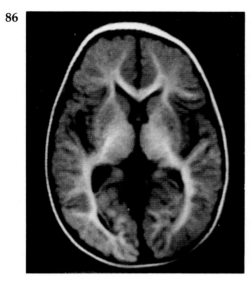

87

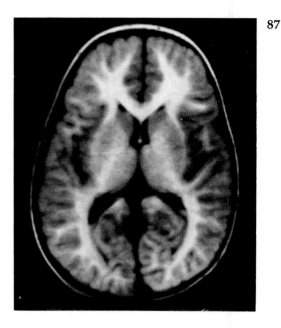

88

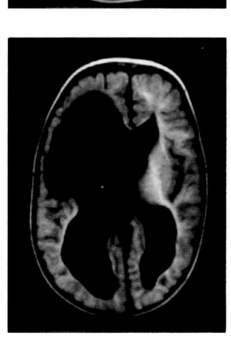

89

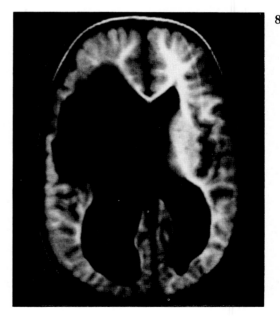

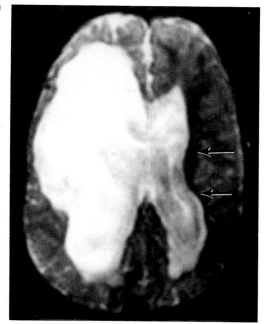

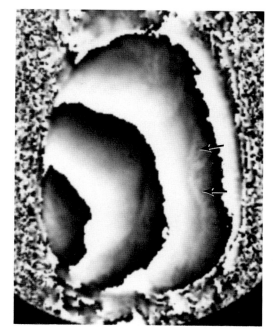

Comment: The marked hemiplegia in the affected twin was expected given the size of the porencephalic cyst. However, she was intellectually intact. It is also of interest that the visual evoked responses did not become asymmetrical until she reached six months of age.

Although there was a delay in myelination in the affected twin compared to her normal sister, the level of white matter development was greater than in case 12 (page 63, figure **126**) who had periventricular leukomalacia as well as intraventricular haemorrhage.

This case illustrates the value of partial saturation sequences and phase mapping for the identification of the breakdown products of old haemorrhage.

Case 10

Premature infant, born at 32 weeks gestation. He developed a large intraventricular and parenchymal haemorrhage in the first week. He had a moderate hemiplegia, but he was intellectually normal. At five years of age he started school and coped well with the normal primary school curriculum.

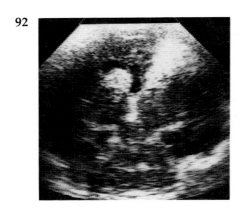

92

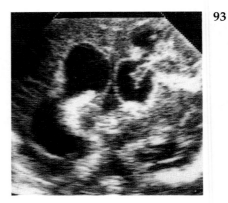

93

Ultrasound: A bilateral intraventricular and a right-sided intraparenchymal haemorrhage occurred on day 2 (**92**), and blood was seen in the third ventricle. The parenchymal lesion evolved into a large porencephalic cyst at the end of the second week (**93**). No other parenchymal lesions were identified on ultrasound.

On day 4, **Auditory Brainstem Evoked Re-sponses** were present at a 90 dB intensity and showed prolonged latencies and poor wave forms (**94**). On day 14 there was a marked improvement in the wave forms, but the I–V interpeak latency was still prolonged. By day 19, the auditory brainstem evoked response was normal, despite marked ventricular dilatation and a porencephalic cyst.

94

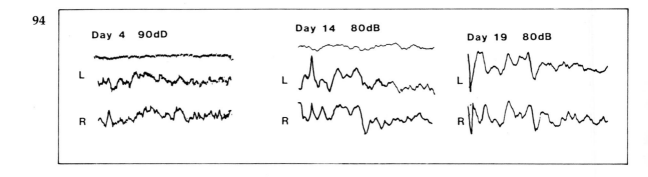

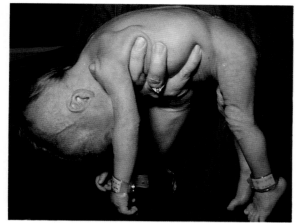

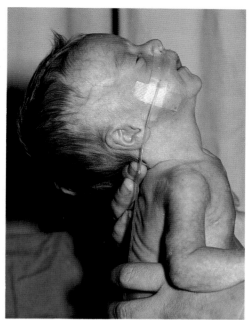

Clinical examination: At 40 weeks postmenstrual age, the child was hypotonic. This is shown in ventral suspension (**95**); however there was some increased extensor tone in the neck (**96**). At six months of age he had remarkably few abnormal signs considering the size of the lesion. Although he did not use his left arm much, only a slight asymmetry of tone could be found on careful neurological examination. He was alert and able to sit with slight support (**97**).

By the end of his first year, the asymmetry in tone was more marked and a hemiplegia was diagnosed, mainly involving his left arm. He had an obvious preference for his right hand (**98**).

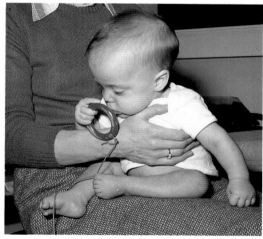

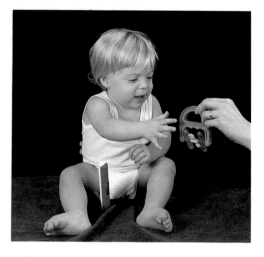

At two years he was able to walk unaided (**99**) and his intellect was normal. At four years he had good coordination in his right hand and could build a tower of eight cubes (**100**).

99

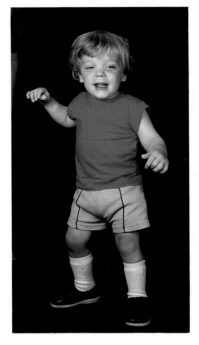

100

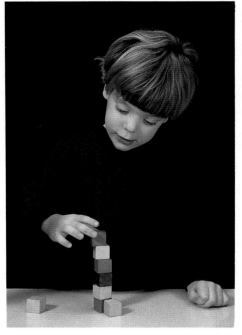

Magnetic Resonance Imaging: Inversion recovery scans are shown at 35 weeks postmenstrual age, 13 months, two years and five years. At 35 weeks postmenstrual age the ventricles were dilated and no white matter was visible. Right frontal and left occipital lobe infarcts were seen as areas of low signal intensity (dark). A large parenchymal haemorrhage was seen on the right with a rim of high signal intensity (bright) surrounding a central core of low signal intensity (dark). A smaller area of haemorrhage (arrow) was seen on the left (**101**). At 13 months the right occipital horn of the lateral ventricle was dilated and myelin was seen in the right hemisphere. Porencephalic cysts had developed at the sites of the previous infarcts (**102**).

101

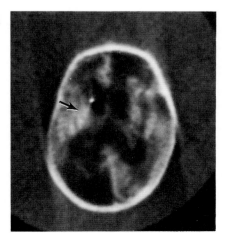

102

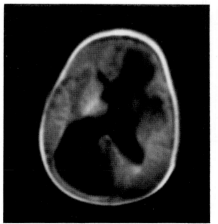

At two years the ventricles were within normal limits and there had been a reduction in the size of the porencephalic cysts. There had been an increase in the level of myelin (**103**). At five years, at a level comparable with **103**, the size and configuration of the ventricles remained unchanged and there had been further progression in myelination (**104**).

103

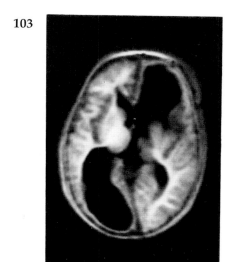

104

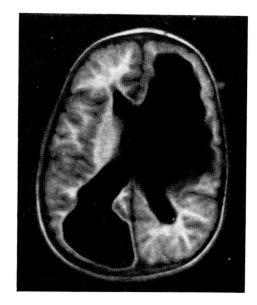

Comment: The left occipital infarct was missed on ultrasound. This may have been due to the poorer resolution of the older scanners, or the lesion may have been too posterior for the beam to penetrate. It is also of interest that, although the initial ABR was very abnormal, it became normal fairly rapidly despite the progressive ventricular dilatation. The remarkably good outcome in this child is attributed to the corresponding contralateral normal areas.

Case 11

Premature infant, born at 26 weeks gestation. She developed a large intraventricular haemorrhage, with parenchymal involvement. She had a marked hemiplegia and visual deficit, but a normal intellect at three years of age.

Ultrasound: The first examination at eight weeks showed a markedly enlarged right ventricle, with a midline shift (**105**). A ventriculo–peritoneal shunt was inserted and the ventricular system collapsed (**106**).

105

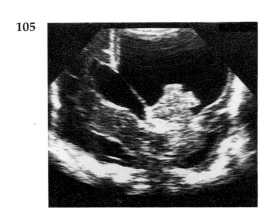

106

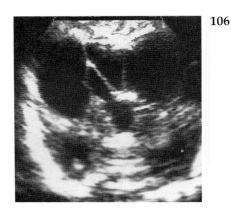

107

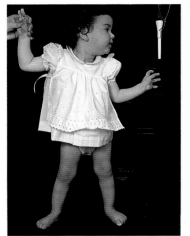

R

L

15 uV

1 sec

Visual Evoked Responses at 40 weeks of age were asymmetrical with poor response on the right (**107**).

Clinical examination: At 15 months of age she sat without support (**108**), could stand with slight support, and had a preference for her right hand (**109**).

108

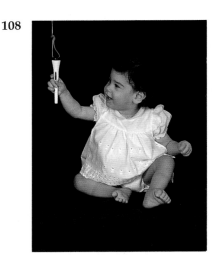

109

At three years she spoke three languages and was able to build a tower of nine bricks (**110**). She used her left hand when necessary, but was clumsy with it (**111**).

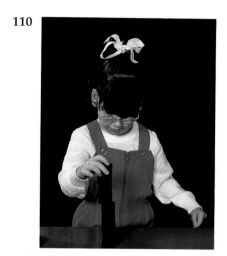

110

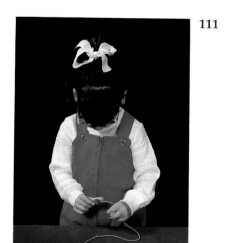

111

Magnetic Resonance Imaging: Inversion recovery scans at two levels are shown at 16 months of age. The right hemisphere was smaller than the left, there was a midline shift, and the right ventricle was enlarged and distorted. No myelin was seen in the right hemisphere but the white matter was within normal limits on the left. A shunt artefact is seen on the right (arrow) (**112**). At the level of the centrum semiovale (**113**) the small and distorted right hemisphere is clearly contrasted with the normal left side.

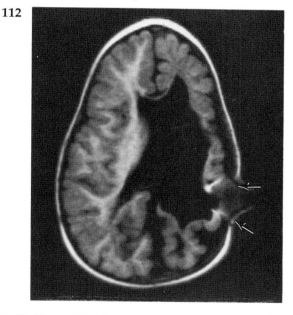

112

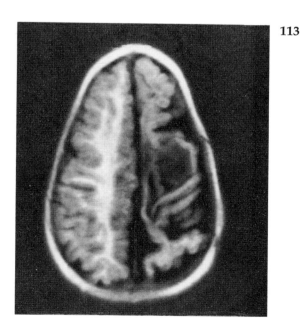

113

Comment: This case illustrates that, even in a very severe form of parenchymal involvement, with extensive destruction of one hemisphere, motor and mental development can be much better than expected. This could be explained by the fact that the insult occurred in a very immature brain, when compensation is more likely to occur.

Case 12

Premature infant, born at 28 weeks gestation, who developed severe hyaline membrane disease. He collapsed on day 2, with pallor, seizures, severe hypotension, hypoxia and a bulging fontanelle. A large intraventricular haemorrhage was diagnosed with associated periventricular leukomalacia. He developed cerebral palsy and hypsarrythmia, and was severely mentally retarded at 12 months, with only slight improvement by four years of age.

Ultrasound examination, after the collapse, showed large ventricular casts and extensive areas of increased echogenicity around the ventricles (**114**) (arrows). Marked ventricular dilatation developed over the next two weeks. A parasagittal view showed a resolving clot in the ventricle and the breakdown of the echogenic area around the occipital horn into cystic lesions (**115**).

114

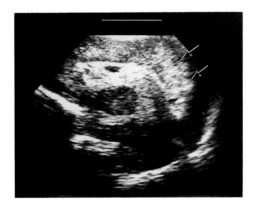

115

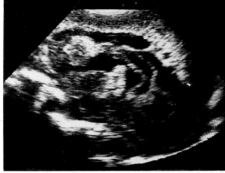

116

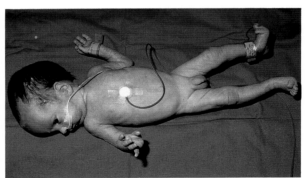

Clinical examination at 36 weeks showed increased arm flexion and leg extension when lying supine; there was also spontaneous extension of the big toes (**116**). In ventral suspension, some leg elevation was present but the head was below the plane of the body (**117**). The progressive ventricular dilatation was accompanied by an increase in head circumference, and the infant was shunted at

117

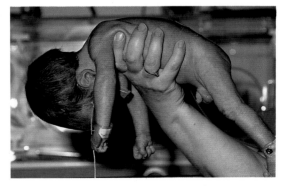

seven months of age. Following the onset of hypsar-rythmia at six months a marked change in tone pattern was seen and he became very hypotonic. At 18 months he had a squint, abnormal eye movements, and no visual orientation could be elicited (**118**). He was unable to sit or to keep his head in line with his body when pulled to sit (**119**) or to sit without support (**120**). He was also severely mentally retarded. Although there was no marked reduction in ventricular size after shunt revision at three years of age, there was some improvement in motor and mental development (**121**).

118

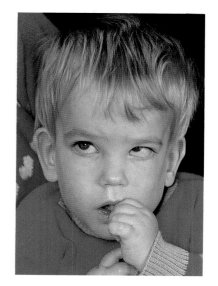

119

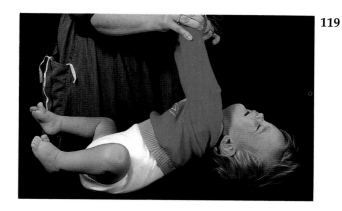

120

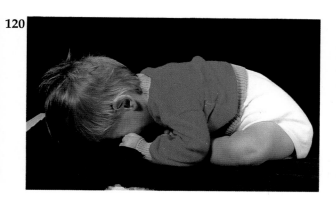

121

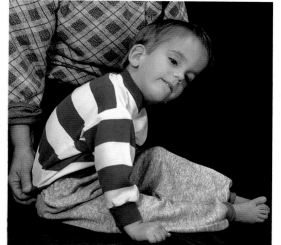

Magnetic Resonance Imaging studies are shown at 2, 12, 24 and 40 months of age. The inversion recovery sequence at two months showed marked dilatation of the posterior horns of the lateral ventricles, and an area of low signal intensity (arrows) was visible within the right occipital pole (**122**). The area of low signal intensity anteriorly on the right (arrow) was due to partial volume effect from the orbit. On the inversion recovery scan at 12 months the ventricles remained dilated despite the shunt (**123**). At two years of age, the ventricles were still dilated and only small amounts of myelin were seen on the inversion recovery scan (**124**). The corresponding short TI inversion recovery sequence showed modest periventricular changes (**125**) compared with the infants with primary but more extensive leukomalacia, for example, Chapter 3, case 12 (page 97).

122

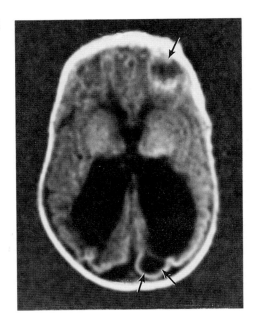

123

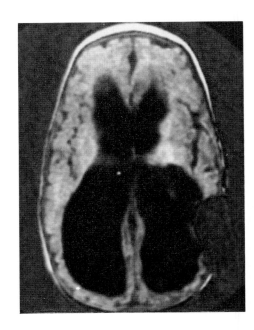

124

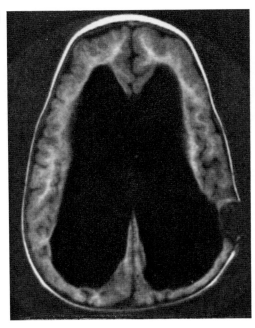

125

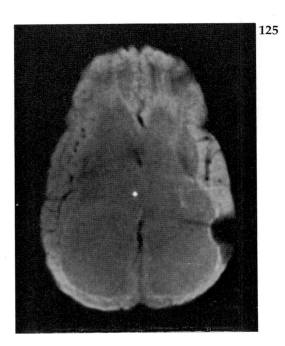

At 40 months, after further shunt revision, the inversion recovery sequence showed a slight decrease in the size of the ventricles but little increase in myelination (**126**). The short TI inversion recovery sequence showed high signal intensity (bright) changes in the periventricular regions, particularly on the left (**127**).

126

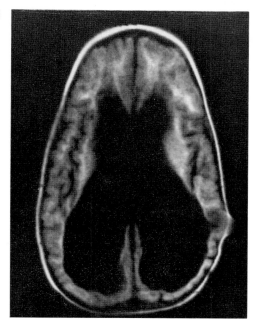

127

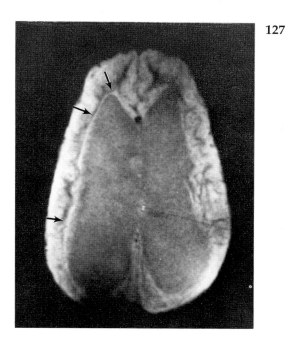

Comment: It is of interest to contrast the outcome of this child with the previous eight cases. Until recently his poor outcome might have been explained by the persistent ventricular enlargement, but it is more likely that the poor outcome was related to the associated bilateral ischaemic lesions. In the neonatal period, some of the clinical signs were more typical of periventricular leukomalacia than intraventricular haemorrhage. The gross delay in myelination may have been due to the periventricular leukomalacia in association with the intraventricular haemorrhage.

Only a few of our premature infants who survived with a large intraventricular or parenchymal haemorrhage have been discussed in this chapter. 45% of our survivors with this type of lesion did not develop any major neurological abnormalities and only 17% had severe handicap with mental retardation (DQ<70, uncorrected for prematurity).

Intraventricular haemorrhage occurs most frequently in very immature infants. However, it can occasionally be seen in full term infants. This is illustrated in the following two cases.

Case 13

Male infant, born at 40 weeks gestation by vaginal vertex delivery. The cord was tightly around his neck and had to be cut before the delivery of his body. His condition was good at birth with Apgar scores of 9 at one and five minutes. At 24 hours of age he had several dusky episodes and was febrile. He was irritable on admission to the neonatal unit.

Electroencephalogram: Continuous 4-channel EEG recording on day 2 was normal (**128**).

An **Ultrasound** scan showed intraventricular haemorrhage on the right (**129**). No ventricular dilatation developed, but the ventricles were prominent at eight months (**130**).

128

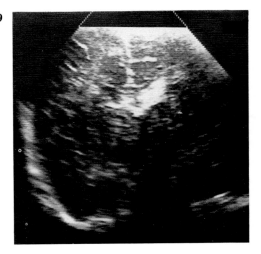

129

130

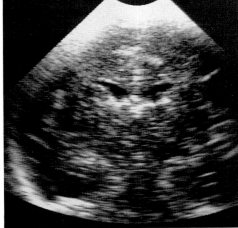

Clinical examination: During the neonatal period he was hypotonic but this resolved during his first year. He was normal at two years except for a delay in speech development. He walked well and played stooping on the floor (**131**). He coped with puzzles appropriate for his age (**132**).

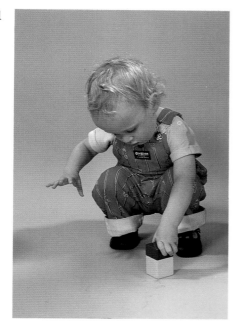

131

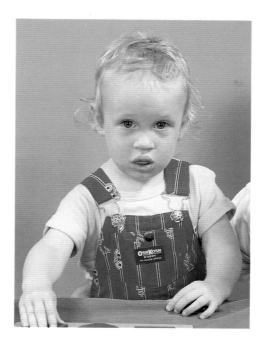

132

Comment: Irritability, seizures and a raised temperature can be the only presenting signs of intraventricular haemorrhage in term infants.

Case 14

Male infant, born by spontaneous vaginal delivery at 38 weeks gestation. Meconium stained liquor was noted before delivery. Apgar scores were 6 and 9 at one and five minutes respectively. He became increasingly jittery over the first 24 hours, which was thought to be due to polycythaemia. At 18 hours of age he had a generalised convulsion. On his second day he was pyrexial with a temperature of 38°C and his fontanelle was full.

Ultrasound examination following admission on day 3 showed bilateral intraventricular haemorrhage, more marked on the left, and an area of increased echogenicity around the external angle of the left ventricle (**133**). Posthaemorrhagic ventricular dilatation developed over the next few weeks (**134**), and the left ventricle was slightly bigger than the right. A ventriculo–peritoneal shunt was inserted at three months of age, and the ventricles decreased in size. A repeat scan at six months of age showed only minimal ventricular dilatation without any evidence of asymmetry (**135**).

133   **134**   **135**

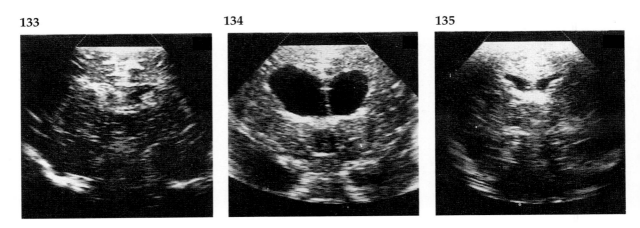

136

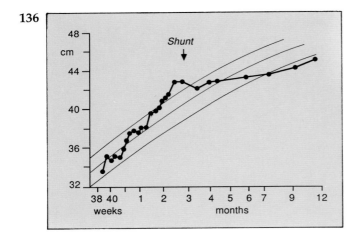

His head circumference increased rapidly prior to shunt insertion at three months of age and a marked decrease was seen after the shunt was inserted. There was no increase in head circumference between four and seven months, and from that time growth continued below but parallel to the 10th centile (**136**).

Auditory Brainstem Evoked Responses were done at 10 days and three months, and at one month after the shunt. They showed a marked deterioration before a shunt was inserted. At this time the intracranial pressure was slightly raised (12 mmHg). A marked improvement in ABR was seen after insertion of the shunt (**137**).

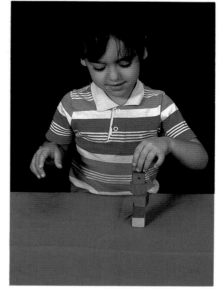

Clinical examination: At the time of admission the infant was very irritable and jittery. He also had a very variable tone pattern but showed persistently more tone in the left arm and left leg compared to the right side; however, his head deviated to the right. By the age of three months his tone pattern had changed; the head was central, his tone was now relatively increased on the right, more in the leg than in the arm. He also had a tight popliteal angle on the right. This pattern persisted. At three years of age he had no severe neurological abnormalities. He walked well (**138**) and used both hands well (**139**).

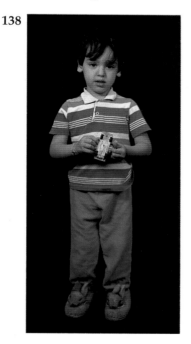

Magnetic Resonance Imaging: inversion recovery images are shown at four and 10 months of age. At the age of three months, and one day after the shunt was inserted the ventricles were dilated (**140**) and very little white matter was seen. Areas of low signal intensity (dark) were visible around the anterior horns of the lateral ventricles (arrows). At 10 months the ventricles were within normal limits. The myelination was slightly delayed. The low signal areas anteriorly persisted (**141**). The shunt tract was clearly seen on this image (arrow).

140

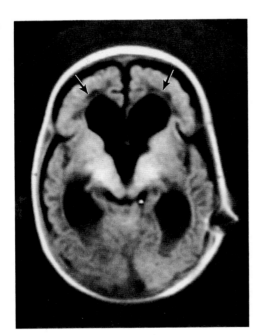

141

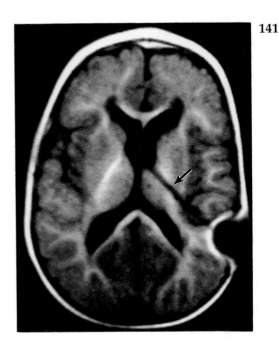

Comment: These two cases, 13 and 14, illustrate intraventricular haemorrhage in term infants. The presenting symptoms may not be very specific and it is worthwhile performing ultrasound scans on all full term infants admitted to an intensive care unit.

Although the initial sequelae to haemorrhage were very different in these two infants, the outcome was favourable in both.

Note also that, while increased intracranial pressure does not have an effect on the auditory brainstem evoked response of premature infants, it is more likely to be abnormal in older infants when the skull is less pliable.

It is also of interest that, in Case 14, the ventricles were still large two days after the shunt was inserted, but the ventricles decreased without any further intervention.

Chapter 3. Leukomalacia

Historical Background

This condition was first described by Virchow in 1867, but the name periventricular leukomalacia was introduced by Banker and Larroche in 1962.

Pathological Features

The pathological features depend on the time that elapses between the onset of the lesion and the time of examination. Coagulation necrosis characterised by loss of normal architectural structure can occur within a few hours. Nuclear debris, astrocytes and macrophages can fill the periphery of the necrotic area within a few days. Liquefaction, resulting in small cavities, can occur in infants who survive for a longer time. The cysts may resolve, leaving areas of gliosis in the otherwise thin periventricular white matter.

Clinical Recognition

Ultrasound is the best imaging modality to identify both the early (echogenic phase) as well as the late changes (cystic phase). The different stages can only be identified on sequential scans. Small cysts (>2 mm) can be identified using a high resolution transducer (7.5 MHz). The appearance of extensive cystic leukomalacia can be subdivided into periventricular, subcortical and mixed, depending on the distribution of the cystic lesions within the cerebral hemispheres.

Periventricular cystic leukomalacia is diagnosed when the cysts are present in the frontal, parietal or occipital periventricular white matter (**1** coronal, **4** parasagittal).

Subcortical cystic leukomalacia is diagnosed when the cysts are present in subcortical white matter (**2** coronal, **5** parasagittal).

Mixed cystic leukomalacia is diagnosed when the features of both the above distributions are present and includes cases in which the cysts are intermediate in position between periventricular and subcortical regions (**3** coronal, **6** parasagittal).

1

2

3

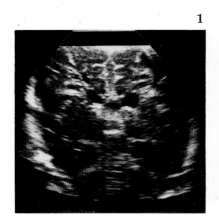
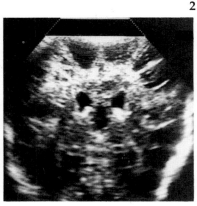
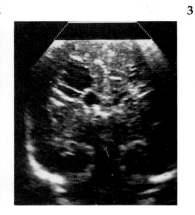

4

5

6

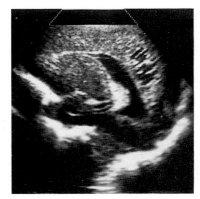

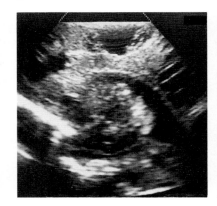

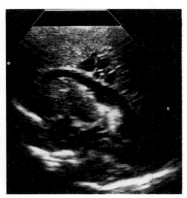

Magnetic Resonance Imaging (MRI) is useful for following the progress in myelination and change in the cystic lesions after closure of the fontanelle. It may be of most value in making the diagnosis of cystic leukomalacia retrospectively in patients who have not had a neonatal ultrasound examination or in whom only some of the classical features have been seen on clinical examination.

X-ray Computed Tomography (CT) examination is useful in the early stages for distinguishing haemorrhagic lesions from nonhaemorrhagic lesions. However, it is not particularly useful in the cystic phase, as only the extensive cystic changes can be seen. Later on, irregularly shaped ventricles might be suggestive of previous cystic lesions.

Clinical examination: preterm infants who develop extensive cystic lesions are often excessively hypotonic in the early stages of the condition. By 40 weeks postmenstrual age they become increasingly hypertonic and are usually extremely irritable.

The change in tone pattern is illustrated in a child of 31 weeks gestation who developed periventricular leukomalacia at birth. She was examined at 33 and 37 weeks postmenstrual age. At her first examination the posture of her legs was normal but there was increased flexion of the arms in the supine position (**7**). Four weeks later there was still increased flexion of the arms (**8**), but now marked extension of the legs was present. On initial examination head lag was noted when she was pulled to sit (**9**), but her head control was much better at 37 weeks postmenstrual age (**10**), and there was also spontaneous extension of the big toe on the left. Her posture in ventral suspension changed considerably. Initially there was excessive trunk and neck hypotonia for this postmenstrual age (**11**). On re-examination, her trunk tone had improved but her head control was too good for this age, suggesting excessive extensor tone (**12**). When held in the sitting position, initially she did not attempt to raise her head (**13**), which was normal for this age. However, at 37 weeks postmenstrual age there was increased neck extensor tone and it was difficult to bring her head forwards (**14**).

7

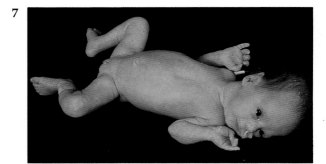

8

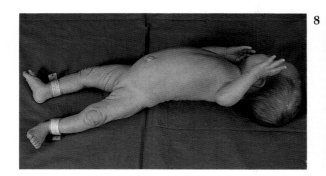

9
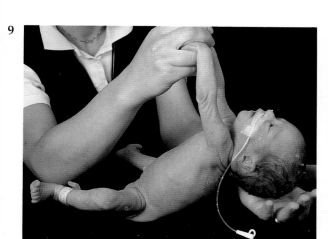

10
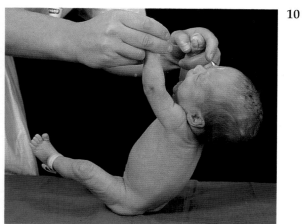

11
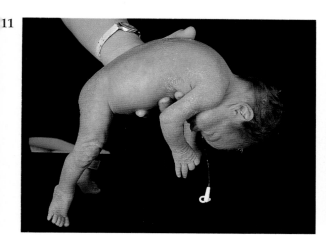

12
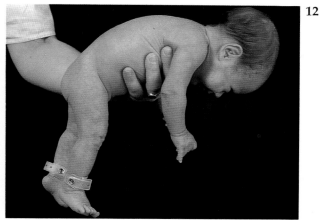

13
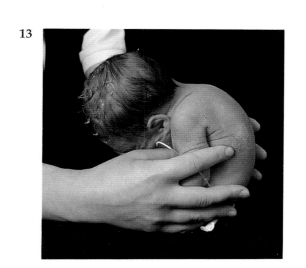

14
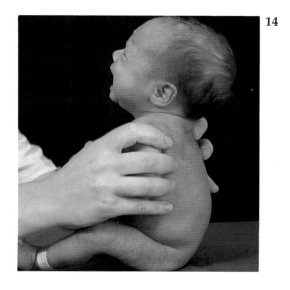

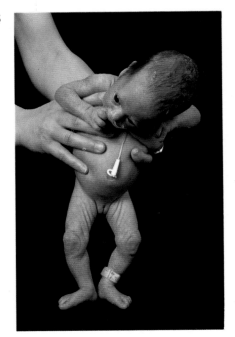

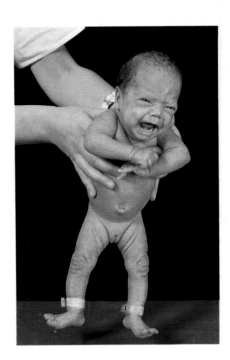

There was also marked change when she was held in a standing position. On initial examination, her head flopped forwards and her legs were slightly flexed (**15**). Four weeks later there was marked extension of the legs and flexion of the arms, and she held her head upright (**16**). Throughout the second examination, at 37 weeks, she was very irritable.

Electrophysiological Tests

Auditory Brainstem Evoked Responses (ABR) are generally of little predictive value and are often completely normal in infants with extensive cystic leukomalacia, particularly after the first week of life. However, in extensive subcortical leukomalacia, an abnormal ratio between wave I and V is often seen in the early stages, and this has been described as an indicator for poor prognosis.

Visual Evoked Responses (VER) are usually present, but sometimes inconsistent, in infants with periventricular cystic leukomalacia; they are normally absent in infants with subcortical leukomalacia.

Somatosensory Potentials tend to be present but delayed in infants with periventricular cystic leukomalacia. They are, however, absent in infants with subcortical leukomalacia.

Electroencephalogram (EEG): continuous four-channel monitoring provides a sensitive index of functional severity of the ischaemic lesions in infants with leukomalacia. Although usually abnormal in infants with periventricular leukomalacia, recovery is seen within a few weeks. However, in infants with subcortical leukomalacia, the abnormalities tend to be much more severe, with low amplitude background and seizure activity. The EEGs of these infants show some improvement with time, but are usually still abnormal at 40 weeks postmenstrual age. In both periventricular and subcortical leukomalacia, EEG abnormalities may precede cyst formation by several weeks and are thus of particular prognostic value.

Case Histories

Cases 1–6 died between three days and three years of age and comparisons were made between the ultrasound scans and the postmortem findings.

Case 1

Premature infant born at 28 weeks gestation. A diaphragmatic hernia was diagnosed at birth, and surgery performed shortly afterwards. Severe hypotension occurred after surgery and the child died at three days of age.

Ultrasound on day 3 showed patchy areas of increased echogenicity adjacent to the lateral ventricles in the coronal (arrows) and parasagittal views (**17** and **18**). An associated intraventricular haemorrhage was also seen in the parasagittal view (**18**).

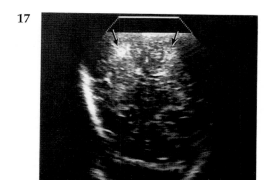

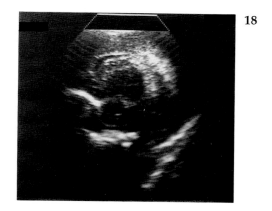

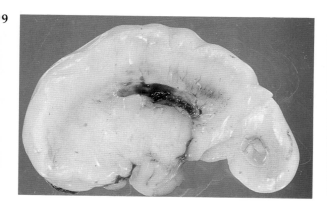

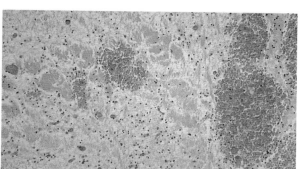

At autopsy the coronal section of the cerebrum showed bilateral subependymal intraventricular haemorrhage with bleeding into periventricular white matter (**19**).

On histology, bleeding into the amorphous pink areas of leukomalacia was seen in the periventricular tissue (Haematoxylin and Eosin × 100) (**20**).

Comment: On macroscopic examination, it was not possible to distinguish between venous infarction and periventricular leukomalacia. However, on histology, changes compatible with periventricular leukomalacia were seen.

Case 2

Premature infant born at 36 weeks gestation. Several dysmorphic features were seen after delivery. Figure **21** shows the infant on the ventilator; note the small lower mandible and the abnormal posture of the fingers (**22**). A complicated heart defect was diagnosed and he died of cardiac failure at 13 days of age. Chromosome studies were normal.

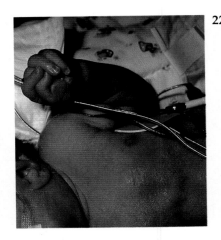

Electroencephalogram: Continuous 4-channel EEG recorded on admission on day 3 showed excessive discontinuity and seizure activity on the right (arrow) (**23**).

The **ultrasound** following admission on day 3 showed diffuse areas of increased echogenicity. The right ventricle could not be seen and appeared compressed (**24**).

At autopsy the coronal section of the cerebrum at the level of the trigone showed pink discoloration of the periventricular tissue.

On histological examination of the periventricular region, a bright pink granular area of degenerating tissue containing a few nuclei was present. This is consistent with early acute periventricular leukomalacia (Haematoxylin and Eosin × 100) (**25**).

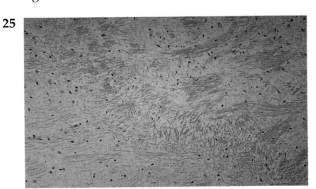

Comment: In case 1, leukomalacia was associated with an intraventricular haemorrhage. In case 2, selective neuronal necrosis was present. These associated findings mainly depend on the maturity of the infant at the time of the insult.

Case 3

Premature infant born at 34 weeks gestation. Initially she had no problems, but deteriorated on day 3 due to cardiac failure and coarctation of the aorta. The coarctation was operated on on day 4 but postoperatively she developed further cardiac and renal failure, and died on day 23.

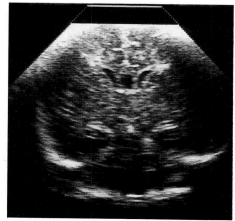

26

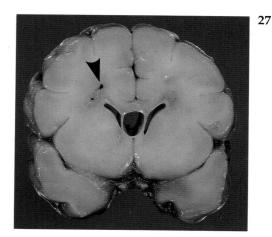

27

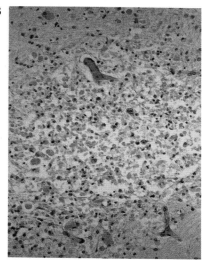

28

Ultrasound examinations were normal until day 5, when areas of increased echogenicity were seen in the periventricular regions. These persisted and a few localised small cysts were seen before death (**26**).

The presence of these small cysts was confirmed at autopsy.

The coronal section of the cerebrum also showed periventricular discoloration with focal haemorrhages and small white spots of periventricular leukomalacia in the right hemisphere (arrow) (**27**).

Histological examination showed a focus of established periventricular leukomalacia, comprising of an area of necrotic tissue infiltrated by macrophages (Haematoxylin and Eosin × 100) (**28**).

Comment: This case illustrates that very small cystic lesions can be confidently identified with ultrasound and that echogenic areas which persist for a long period may represent areas of gliosis.

Case 4

Premature infant, first of twins, born at 30 weeks gestation. She was well until two weeks of age, when she had an acute clinical deterioration. Her ultrasound showed bilateral intraventricular haemorrhages extending into the thalami. Large areas of increased echogenicity were also seen around both lateral ventricles. She later developed extensive cystic leukomalacia and posthaemorrhagic hydrocephalus. A ventriculo–peritoneal shunt was inserted at nine weeks of age, but she died two weeks later.

Ultrasound examinations were completely normal for the first 15 days (**29**). On day 16, large bilateral intraventricular haemorrhages were seen extending into the thalami. The haemorrhage was more extensive on the right (**30**). In addition, large areas of increased echogenicity were seen separate from the ventricles. These were present anterior to the right ventricle on the coronal view with the scanhead angled backwards (**30**), and around both occipital horns (**31** left and **32** right) in the parasagittal view.

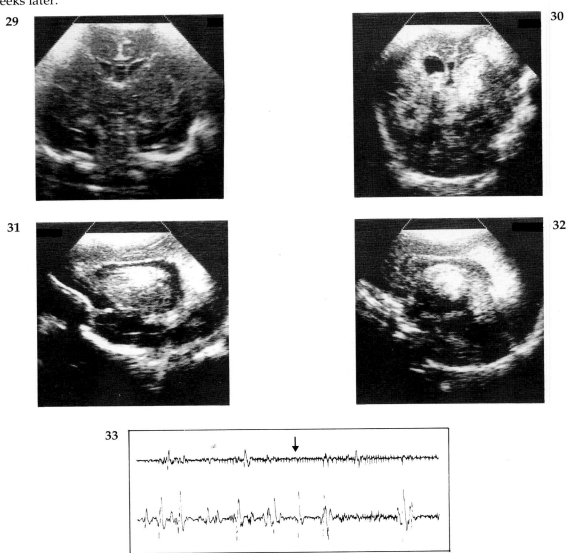

Electroencephalogram: Continuous 4-channel EEG at this time showed excessive discontinuity and seizure activity (arrow). The recording was asymmetrical and asynchronous (**33**).

The echogenic areas broke down into cystic lesions and massive ventricular dilatation occurred. The cystic lesions on the right were initially separate from the lateral ventricle, but communication subsequently occurred (34). The cysts on the left side remained separate from the lateral ventricle (35).

Autopsy confirmed the presence and distribution of the cystic lesions (36). Note that on the parasagittal section of the left hemisphere looking from the lateral aspect towards the foramen of Monro, there were multiple periventricular cysts around the grossly dilated ventricle. On histological examination the wall of the periventricular cyst (to right of picture) showed a small additional area of periventricular leukomalacia with macrophage infiltration (centre left) (37).

34

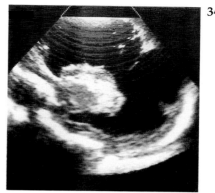

35

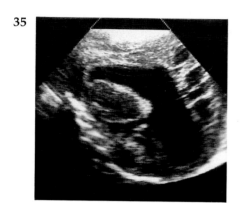

36

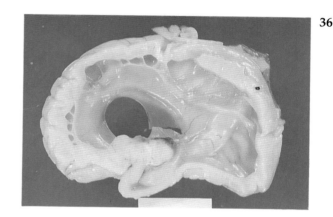

37

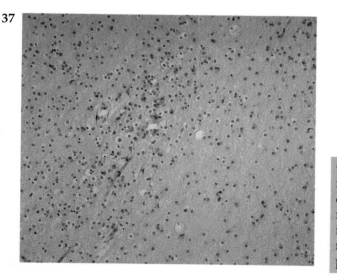

Comment: This case illustrates the progression of ischaemic lesions to cyst formation, and how breakdown of the ventricular wall may lead to communication with the ventricular cavity. If the first scan is done at the time this occurs, the lesion might be misdiagnosed as a porencephalic cyst following a parenchymal haemorrhage.

Case 5

Premature infant born at 27 weeks gestation. He developed severe respiratory distress syndrome and broncho–pulmonary dysplasia. Apnoeic spells occurred following an attempted extubation at four weeks of age. Periventricular densities were noted at this time, which developed into cystic leukomalacia. At seven months he died of cardio–respiratory failure following a viral infection.

Ultrasound: The coronal and parasagittal views at four weeks of age showed an area of increased echogenicity behind the occipital horn of the lateral ventricle (**38**, **41**). Three weeks later small cystic lesions had developed in the previously echogenic areas (**39**, **42**). At six months the cysts were no longer visible but the left occipital horn was dilated (**40**, **43**).

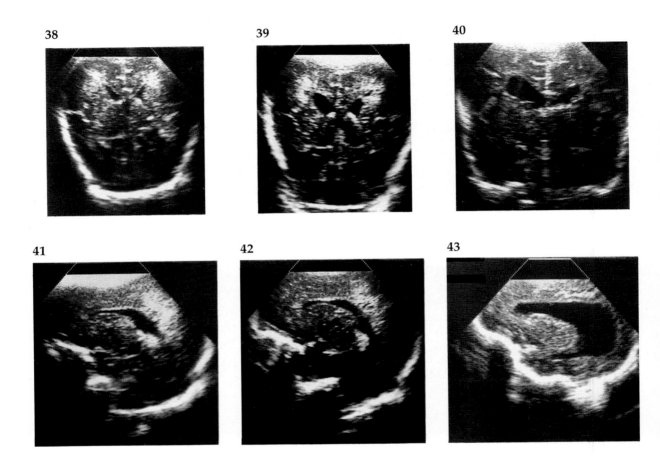

At autopsy, the coronal section of the occipital lobe showed a mildly dilated ventricle and poor myelination, but no cystic lesions were seen on macroscopic examination (**44**).

On histology, the periventricular regions showed an area of gliosis containing lipid filled macrophages (Haematoxylin and Eosin × 100) (**45**).

44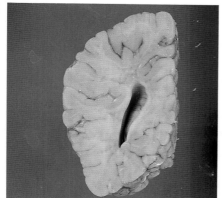

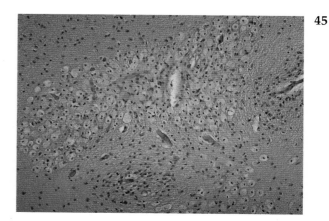 **45**

Comment: This case illustrates that, in the late stages of periventricular leukomalacia, the cysts may completely disappear. The lesions due to leukomalacia can be missed unless histology as well as macroscopic examination are carried out.

Case 6

Premature infant born at 31 weeks gestation. At eight days of age he developed apnoeic spells and required ventilation. A diagnosis of mixed cystic leukomalacia was made. He developed quadriplegia, was severely mentally retarded and cortically blind. He died at three years of age.

Ultrasound: He was referred to our hospital at eight days of age without having had previous ultrasound scans. His first ultrasound showed areas of increased echogenicity around dilated ventricles, with a few cysts in the echogenic areas (**46**). Extensive cystic lesions developed over the next two weeks (**47**). Initially these cysts were separate from the ventricles, but communication subsequently developed and septi were seen, especially on the left (**48**). There was a rapid increase in the size of the ventricles, with a rise in intracranial pressure. A ventriculo–peritoneal shunt was inserted at three months, and the ventricles collapsed.

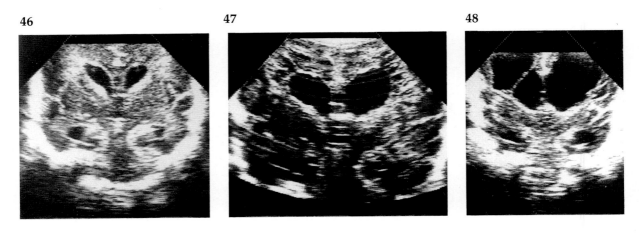

46 47 48

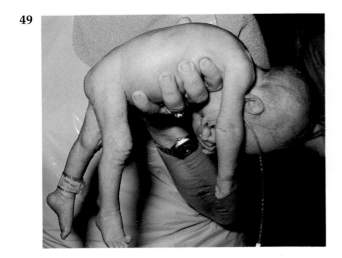

49

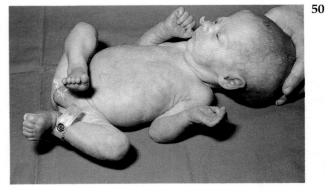

50

Clinical examination: At 40 weeks postmenstrual age the infant was still hypotonic in ventral suspension (**49**) (note the up-going toe on the right).

Supine, he showed normal flexion of his legs but increase in arm flexion for 40 weeks postmenstrual age (**50**).

At 18 months of age, he was severely handicapped and unable to sit without support (**51**).

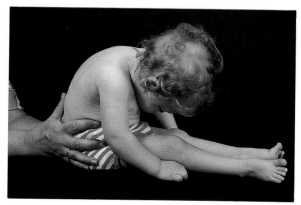

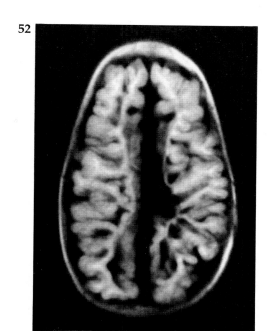

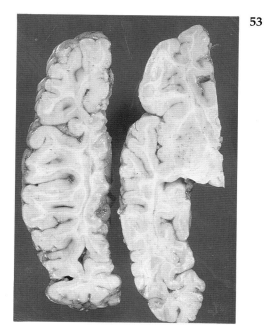

Magnetic Resonance Imaging: The inversion recovery scan at 24 months showed collapsed ventricles and a few fine strands of white matter extending to the cortex. The interhemispheric fissure was widened and the sulci were prominent. Extensive areas of low signal intensity (dark) were seen throughout both hemispheres (**52**).

The gross delay in development of myelination seen with MRI compared well with the myelin seen on the macroscopic section obtained after death at 34 months (**53**).

Comment: In this infant, progressive ventricular dilatation coincided with the breakdown of periventricular cysts. This is unusual in the absence of an associated large intraventricular haemorrhage. As ultrasound studies were not available in the first week of life, it is not known if or when a haemorrhage occurred. Alternatively, the hydrocephalus might have been due to an obstruction caused by broken-down debris.

This case illustrates the excellent correlation between white matter seen on magnetic resonance imaging and macroscopic sections.

The following 13 case reports illustrate the evolution of the lesions and the outcome in infants who survived with extensive cystic leukomalacia.

In cases 7–12, periventricular leukomalacia was diagnosed in the early neonatal period with ultrasound, whereas cases 13, 14 and 15 were diagnosed on clinical examination at a time when adequate ultrasound was no longer possible. In these latter, the diagnosis could be confirmed with magnetic resonance imaging.

Cases 16 and 17 are examples of mixed cystic leukomalacia, and cases 18 and 19 of subcortical cystic leukomalacia.

Cases 20 and 21 describe the outcome in twins, one with an intraventricular haemorrhage and the other with periventricular leukomalacia.

Periventricular leukomalacia

Case 7

Premature infant born at 30 weeks gestation, with a birth weight of 840 grams (<3rd centile). He developed severe respiratory distress syndrome and broncho–pulmonary dysplasia. Marked periventricular densities were first noted following treatment with dexamethasone at three weeks of age. Localised cystic leukomalacia occurred, and he later developed transient dystonia.

Ultrasound: Two days after the beginning of dexamethasone the coronal view showed areas of increased echogenicity around the anterior horns of the lateral ventricles (**54**) (arrow). Three weeks later a few localised cysts were seen in the echogenic areas. The cysts were only present anteriorly on the coronal (**55**) and parasagittal views (**56**) (arrows). At six months there was some widening of the interhemispheric fissure (**57**).

54
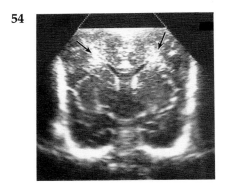

55
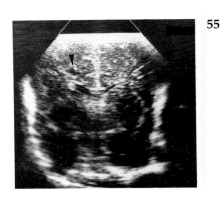

56
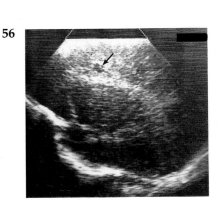

57
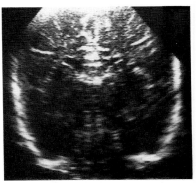

Clinical examination: At 12 months the child was bright (**58**) but hyperactive. There was a delay in motor milestones and his popliteal angles were tight (**59**). At 15 months he was able to pull himself into a standing position but could not stand without support (**60**). He walked at 22 months.

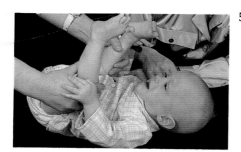

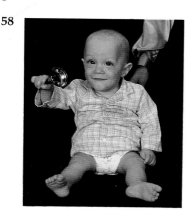

Magnetic Resonance Imaging: At 15 months the inversion recovery sequence through the centrum semiovale showed low signal intensity areas (dark) in the white matter anteriorly (arrows) (**61**). These lesions were seen as high signal intensity areas (bright) on the short TI inversion recovery scan at the same level (**62**).

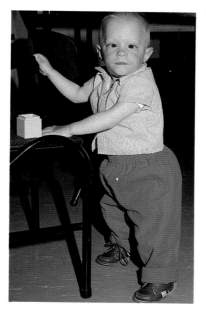

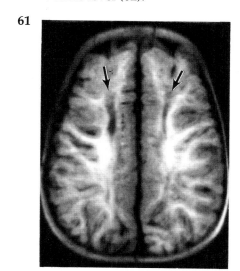

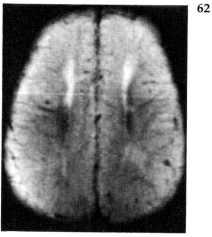

Comment: This case illustrates the expected outcome in a child when the cystic lesions are confined to the anterior part of the centrum semiovale. In the majority of infants with anterior periventricular densities, the densities disappear without evolving into cysts. Motor signs are present during the first 6–12 months in the majority of children, but they become normal later. If a follow-up clinical examination had been performed after the first year, it may have been concluded that this milder type of lesion had no adverse effect at all. However, as these children tend to develop problems at school, recognition is important.

Case 8

Premature infant born at 31 weeks gestation. He recovered from moderate respiratory distress syndrome, but at two weeks of age he had a sudden clinical deterioration. He developed bilateral intraventricular haemorrhage associated with periventricular leukomalacia, to be followed, later, by cerebral palsy, infantile spasms and mental retardation.

Initially the **ultrasound** findings were normal. At two weeks of age, after clinical deterioration, a coronal ultrasound showed a bilateral intraventricular haemorrhage extending down into the thalami (arrow), and bilateral areas of increased echogenicity adjacent to the anterior horns of the ventricles (**63**) (arrows). Four weeks later the haemorrhages had resolved and cystic lesions were seen in the previously dense areas (**64**) (arrow). The anterior cysts were seen on the parasagittal image (arrow) but no cysts were seen posteriorly (**65**). Infantile spasms started at four months and marked ventricular dilatation with widening of the interhemispheric fissure was seen at this time (**66**). The third ventricle was also dilated (arrow).

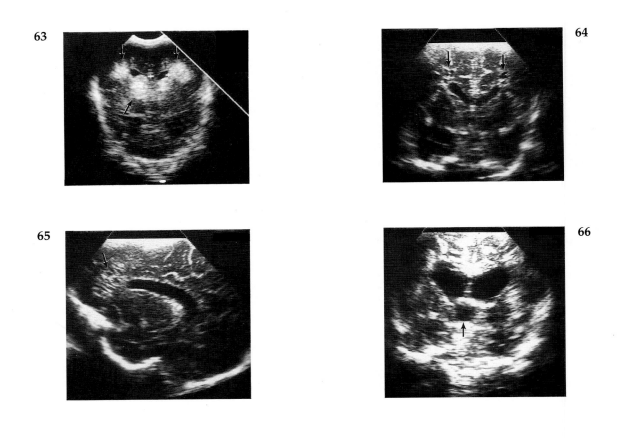

Clinical examination took place at nine months of age, when he was being treated for hypsarrythmia. He showed severe delay in development. Marked head lag was present when he was pulled to sit (**67**), and he was unable to sit without support (**68**). Increased extensor tone of the legs was present in ventral suspension (**69**).

At 12 months a slight improvement was noted and he showed more interest in his surroundings and maintained his head upright for a short time when held in a sitting position (**70**). There was marked tightness of the popliteal angles (**71**) and the lateral tilting reactions were absent (**72**).

67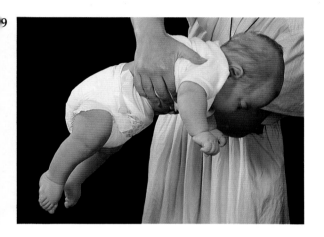

68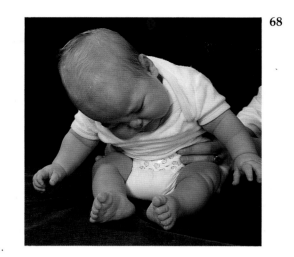

69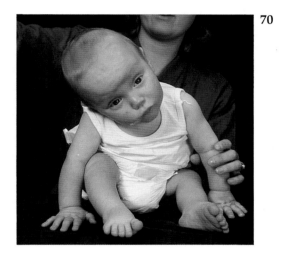

70

71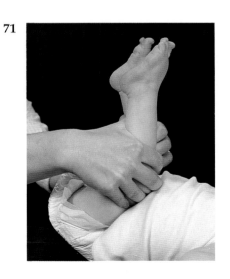

72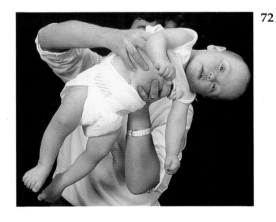

At 20 months, further improvement was seen and he was able to get on to his hands and knees for a short time (73). With help he could also pull himself up to a standing position (74). However, his popliteal angles were still very tight (75).

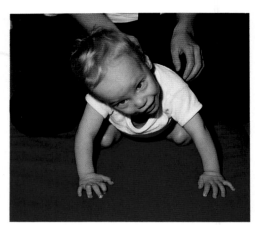

73

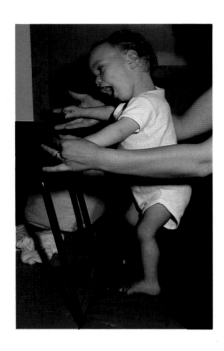

74

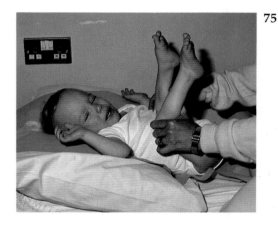

75

Magnetic Resonance Imaging: At 11 months the inversion recovery scan showed ventricular dilatation which was more marked anteriorly. The posterior horns were irregular and sharply angled. There was widening of the interhemispheric fissure and the sulci were prominent. Only fine strands of myelin were identified (76). The partial saturation image showed low signal intensity areas in the periventricular regions (arrows) (77) and around the sulci, with corresponding susceptibility changes (arrows) (78) indicating the presence of old haemorrhage. At 18 months the ventricular system was unchanged in shape but there was some progression in myelination, especially posteriorly on the right (79). At a low ventricular level the myelination was delayed (80).

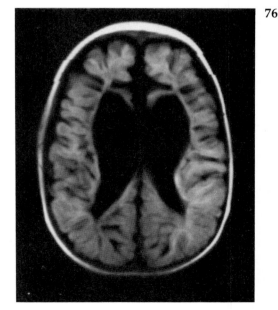

76

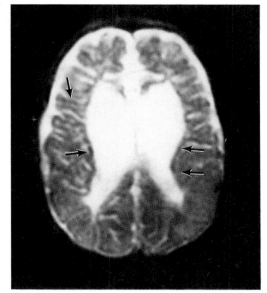

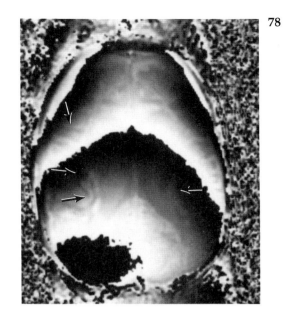

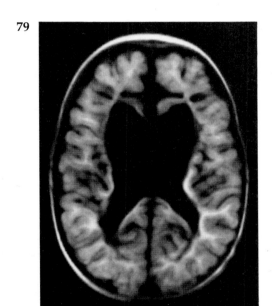

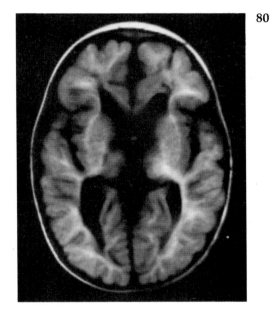

Comment: This case raises an interesting point. His cysts were located anteriorly and he showed few deviant neurological signs at 40 weeks postmenstrual age. However, following the onset of infantile spasms, a marked deterioration occurred in his motor and mental performances, and a change of tone pattern was also observed. He became severely hypotonic before any treatment was started. Infants with anterior lesions appear to be more likely to develop infantile spasms, and their poor development may be closely related to this severe complication.

The value of susceptibility mapping for old haemorrhage is well demonstrated in this infant. Haemorrhage may appear as high signal (bright) on the inversion recovery sequence and may be difficult to distinguish from myelin. Susceptibility mapping will help to solve this problem.

Case 9

Premature infant born at 30 weeks gestation. He recovered from a moderate respiratory distress syndrome but there was a clinical deterioration at two weeks of age, for which no explanation was found. He sustained bilateral intraventricular haemorrhages and associated cystic periventricular leukomalacia. He had spastic diplegia, and a mild to moderate mental retardation.

Ultrasound: The studies were normal until he developed apnoeic spells and seizures on day 15. A coronal view with the scan head angled backwards showed bilateral intraventricular haemorrhage (arrow) and areas of increased echogenicity adjacent to the lateral ventricles (**81**) (arrows). These findings could have been confused with 'parenchymal extension' but a **CT** scan done two days later (**82**) showed areas of increased attenuation inside the lateral ventricles, but no areas of increased attenuation in the periventricular regions.

Three weeks later the haemorrhages had resolved, but cystic lesions were present in the previously echogenic periventricular areas (**83**) (arrows). In the parasagittal view the cystic lesions were mainly confined to the anterior and parietal periventricular regions (**84**).

Magnetic Resonance Imaging: The inversion recovery scan at 35 weeks showed extensive areas of low signal intensity in the centrum semiovale (**85**).

81

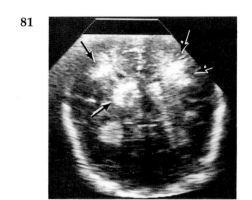

82

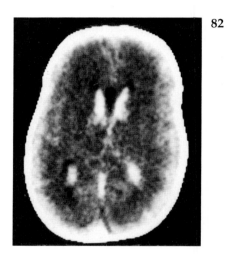

83

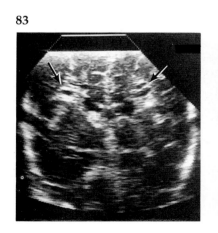

84

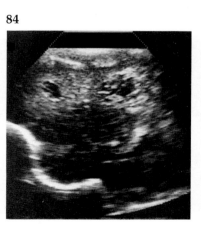

85

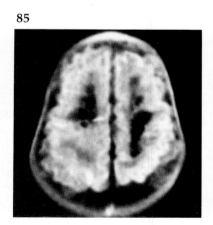

Clinical examination: At nine months of age he showed marked tightening of the popliteal angles (**86**). At 12 months he stood with support (**87**), but there was increased extensor tone (**88**). At two and a half years he could not stand without support and still showed increased extensor tone (**89**). He developed convulsions at three years of age and there was considerable deterioration in his concentration and hand manipulation. He had marked difficulty threading beads (**90**).

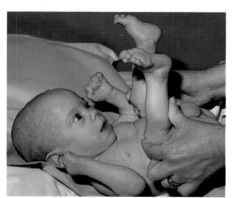

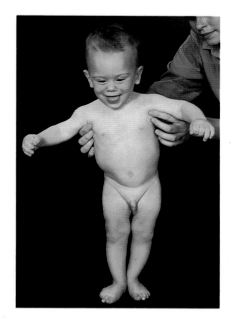

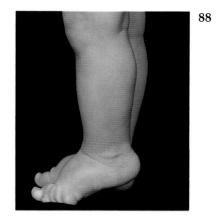

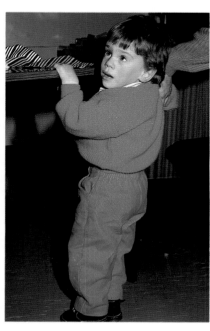

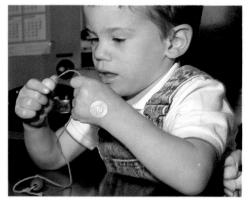

Magnetic Resonance Imaging: At eight months the ventricles were within normal limits and there was a delay in myelination, especially anteriorly (**91**). Areas of low signal intensity were also seen anteriorly (arrows) on the inversion recovery sequence. At 21 months of age there had been an increase in the level of myelination, especially posteriorly, and the low signal intensity areas were still present around the anterior horns on the inversion recovery sequence (**92**). Corresponding areas of high signal intensity were seen on the short TI inversion recovery sequence (arrows) (**93**).

91

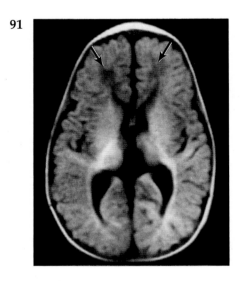

92

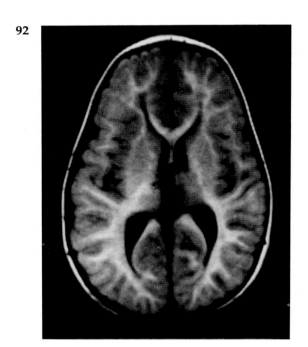

93

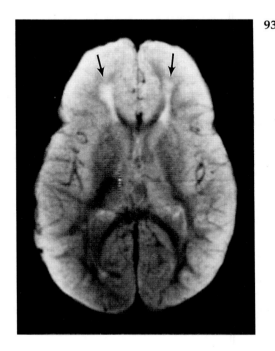

Comment: This case illustrates that the distinction between haemorrhagic and non-haemorrhagic periventricular leukomalacia cannot be made with ultrasound. It can, however, be made if a CT scan is done within seven days of the onset of the haemorrhage. At this stage the haemorrhage appears as an area of high attenuation. After seven days the lesion will be isodense with the brain.

Although cystic lesions were mainly in the frontal and parietal areas, he did not develop hypsarrythmia. At three years of age, however, he developed seizures, following which there was considerable clinical deterioration.

Case 10

Premature infant born at 29 weeks gestation. During the first 24 hours he was ventilated for six hours following an apnoeic spell. He required further ventilation for 48 hours in the second week for recurrent apnoea. Areas of increased echogenicity were seen during the second period of ventilation. At follow-up this child had spastic diplegia and was able to walk at three and a half years of age. His intellect was normal.

Ultrasound examinations in the first week were normal but his **electroencephalogram** showed discontinuity and seizure activity (**94**) (arrow).

During the second period of ventilation, areas of increased echogenicity were seen around the ventricles in the coronal view with the scan head angled backwards (**95**), and around the occipital horns in the parasagittal view (**96**). The echogenic areas persisted for four weeks, but no cystic lesions were seen.

94
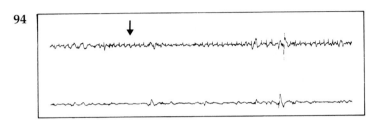

95
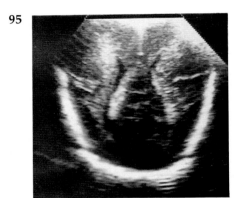

96
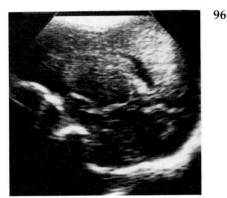

Clinical examination: At nine months of age he showed signs of spastic diplegia and there was tightness of the popliteal angles (**97**). He had a marked tendency to scissor when held in a standing position (**98**). He had a mild squint, but no visual deficit.

98
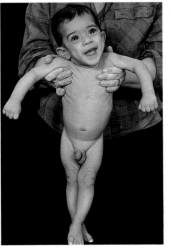

97
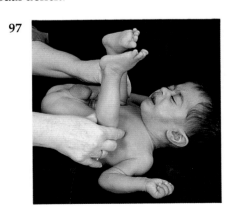

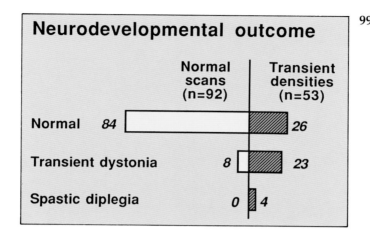

99

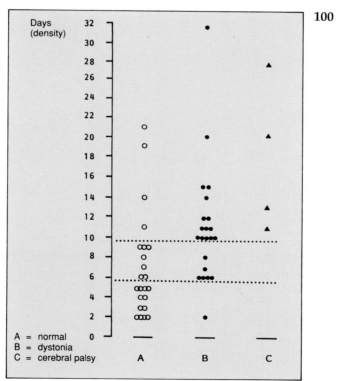

100

Infants with transient densities are more likely to develop transient dystonia compared to infants with normal scans. Of 92 infants with completely normal scans, 84 had a normal outcome. Less than 10% had dystonia and none had cerebral palsy, while more than half the infants with densities had later abnormalities (**99**). Cerebral diplegia is a relatively uncommon sequela and seems to be associated particularly with occipital densities.

The abnormalities are particularly common when the densities persist for 10 days or more (**100**).

Case 11

Premature infant born at 28 weeks gestation by an emergency caesarean section following antepartum haemorrhage. She developed localised cystic leukomalacia and mild spastic diplegia, and was able to walk unaided, albeit with an abnormal gait, at two years of age.

Ultrasound: The scans performed during the first days of life showed bilateral areas of increased echogenicity around the frontal (**101**) and occipital (**102**) horns of the lateral ventricles.

Electroencephalogram: Continuous 4-channel EEG recorded during the first week of life was unequivocally abnormal, with possibly some asymmetry and asynchrony (**103**).

At 31 weeks postmenstrual age a right occipital cyst was seen in the coronal view with the scan head angled backwards (**104**), and in the parasagittal view (**105**) (arrow). The cyst was no longer visible at 38 weeks postmenstrual age. At seven months there was moderate ventricular dilatation.

101

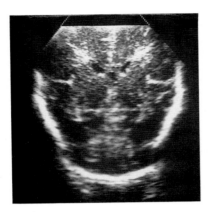

102

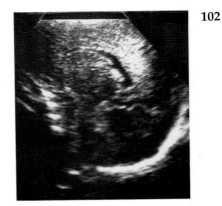

103

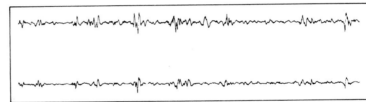

104

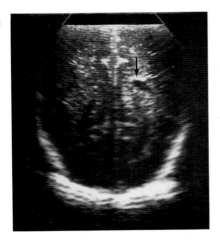

105

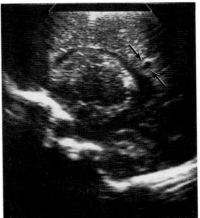

Clinical examination: At seven months she was alert and sociable (**106**). Increased extensor tone was found on careful neurological assessment, when she was held in a standing position (**107**) and in ventral suspension (**108**). Her deviant neurological signs were more marked at 12 months, when she was still unable to roll over or sit without support for longer than a few seconds (**109**). She had a tendency to fall backwards (**110**) and she showed spontaneous extension of the big toe.

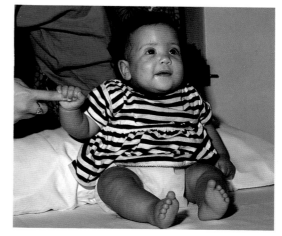

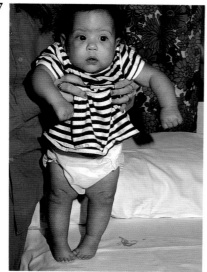

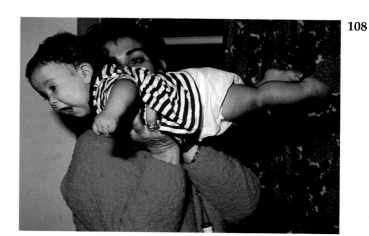

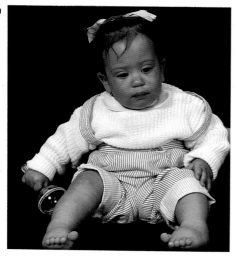

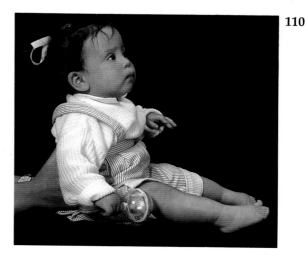

111

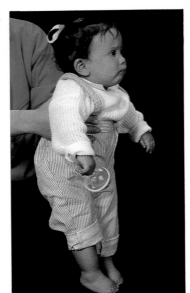

She tended to tiptoe when held in a standing position (111) and her popliteal angles were tight, more so on the left (112).

11?

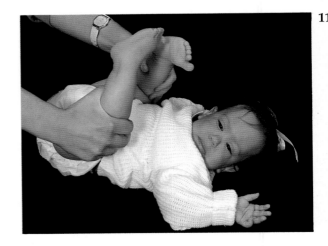

113

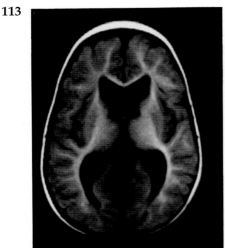

114

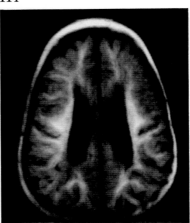

115

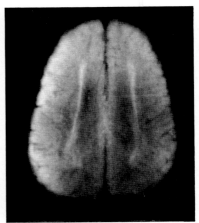

Magnetic Resonance Imaging: At 12 months the inversion recovery scan showed mild ventricular dilatation at a low ventricular level, and myelination was slightly delayed (113). At mid ventricular level there was some delay in myelination, especially posteriorly (114). A short TI inversion recovery sequence at the same level showed areas of high intensity (bright) in the periventricular regions (115).

Comment: This case illustrates that even small lesions in the posterior part of the centrum semiovale are markers for the more persistent motor disturbances. Although the cystic lesions were unilateral the echogenic areas were bilateral. MRI confirmed symmetrical lesions in keeping with her later bilateral deficit.

Case 12

Premature infant born at 27 weeks gestation, with a birth weight of 1190 grams. A diagnosis of cystic periventricular leukomalacia was made at 33 weeks postmenstrual age. Her first assessment at our hospital was at 40 weeks. She later developed spastic diplegia with a normal intellect.

Ultrasound: No early scans were available. At 40 weeks postmenstrual age extensive periventricular cysts were present. The cysts were most marked around the occipital horns (**116**), and were clearly visible in the coronal view with the scan head angled backwards (**117**). The cysts did not communicate with the lateral ventricles.

116

117

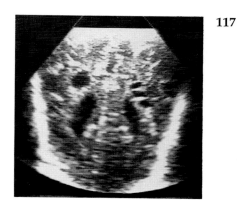

118

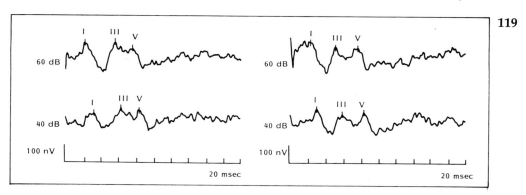

Visual Evoked Responses at 40 weeks showed no positivity, which is a sign of immaturity at this age (**118**).

Auditory Brainstem Evoked Responses at 40 weeks showed normal wave forms and normal latencies at 60 and 40 dB intensity (**119**).

119

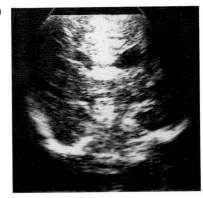

120

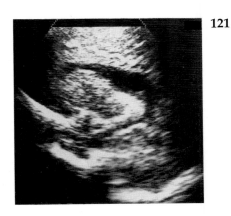

121

At six months of age no cystic lesions were seen, but there was asymmetry in ventricular size (**120**) and irregularly dilated occipital horns (**121**).

Clinical examination: At five months of age she was irritable. She was able to keep her head in the plane of her body when pulled to sit (**122**). There was tightness of the popliteal angles (**123**) and some adductor spasm (**124**). In ventral suspension her legs were elevated but she had good trunk control (**125**).

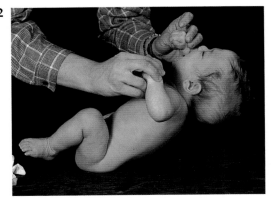

122

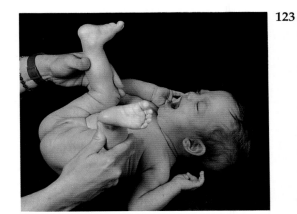

123

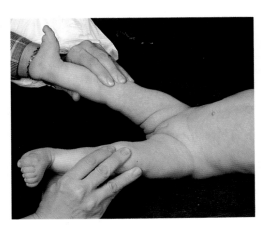

124

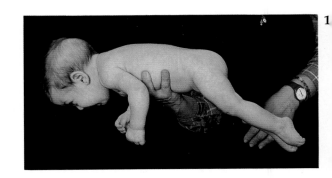

1

At 12 months she was a bright little girl who showed classical signs of spastic diplegia with a marked tendency to scissor (**126**). She had severe alternating strabismus (**127**). Her lateral tilting reflexes were absent (**128**) and she was unable to elevate her legs or head in ventral suspension (**129**). Her popliteal angles remained tight (**130**).

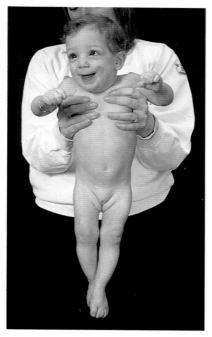

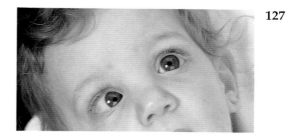

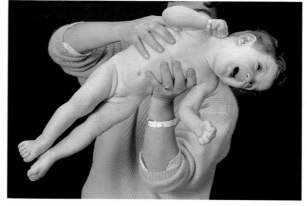

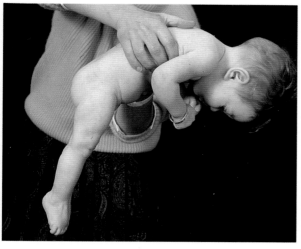

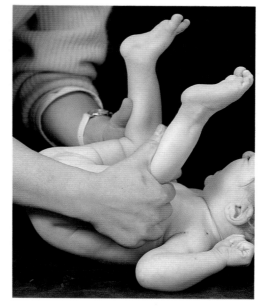

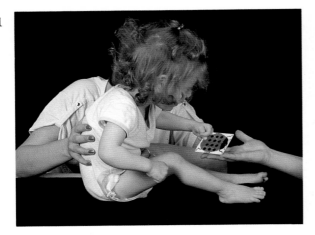

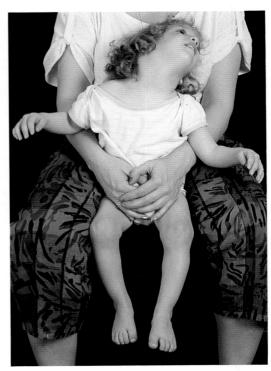

At two years of age she was unable to sit without support and her hand manipulation was poor (**131**). Her trunk control was poor and she tended to fall backwards when held in a sitting position (**132**). She could stand only with considerable support (**133**).

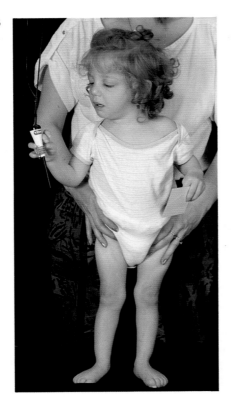

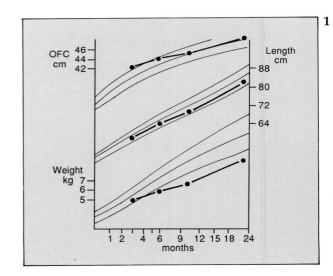

Her head circumference fell from the 90th to the 50th centile between three and 10 months of age, and continued to grow along the 50th centile. Her length and weight also crossed the centiles during the same period (**134**).

Magnetic Resonance Imaging: The inversion recovery scan at nine months of age showed ventricular dilatation, and the occipital horns were irregular and sharply angulated. Myelination was delayed, especially posteriorly (**135**). Extensive high signal intensity areas were seen in the periventricular regions on the short TI inversion recovery sequence (**136**).

A repeat scan at 20 months of age at the same level showed little change in ventricular size and a marked progression in myelination, especially around the anterior horns (**137**).

The high signal intensity areas were present but less obvious on the corresponding short TI inversion recovery scan (**138**).

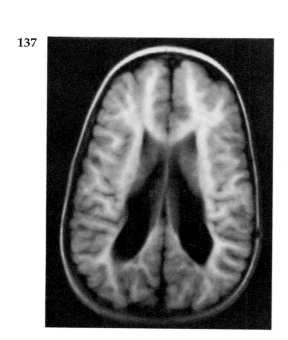

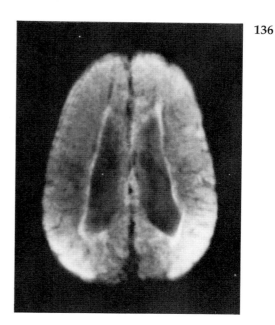

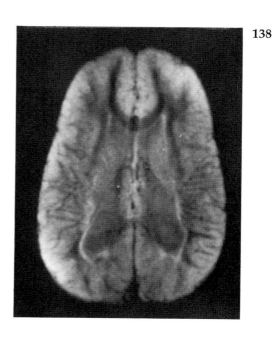

The inversion recovery sequence through the centrum semiovale at 20 months showed bilateral areas of low signal intensity (arrows) (139); these areas were seen more clearly on the corresponding short TI inversion recovery sequence as high signal intensity (140).

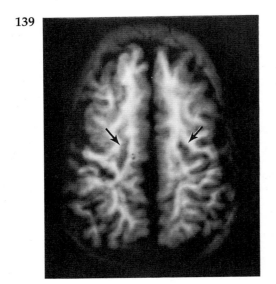

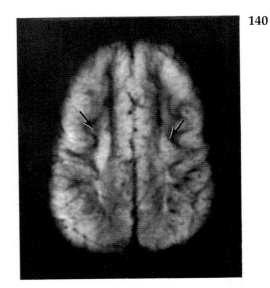

CT at 22 months of age showed irregular lateral ventricles with posterior dilatation (141), and appearances suggestive of cyst formation in the centrum semovale (142) (but this is difficult to distinguish from partial volume effects between brain and cerebrospinal fluid).

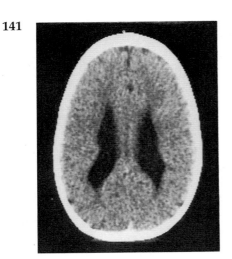

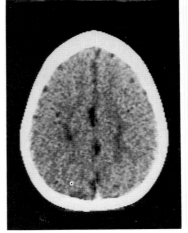

Comment: This case has been reported extensively to show the classical features found in children with periventricular cystic leukomalacia.

With ultrasound, the extensive cysts cannot be seen after four months of age. This is probably due to absorption of the cystic fluid by the surrounding brain tissue. Irregular ventricular dilatation usually occurs at this time.

Ventricular dilatation and irregularly shaped ventricles can be seen on both CT and MRI. However, MRI provides more information. It may show a global delay or deficit in myelination, or a specific delay or deficit at the sites of the cystic lesions. This case also illustrates that good progress in myelination can be seen in the unaffected areas in infants with periventricular cystic leukomalacia.

As myelination progresses, the areas of low signal intensity which correspond to the sites of the cystic lesions seen on ultrasound are more difficult to define on the medium inversion time inversion recovery sequence. This is probably due to partial volume effects. However, the short TI inversion recovery sequence is extremely sensitive to lesions in white matter and in the periventricular regions, and thus highlights the sites of the lesions. Some high signal seen on the short TI inversion recovery

sequence has remained present in our infants at follow-up studies up to four years of age.

It is of interest that the periventricular change seen on the short TI inversion recovery scan in infants with primary cystic leukomalacia was more marked than in the infants whose primary lesion was intraventricular haemorrhage (Chapter 2, case 12).

The visually evoked responses are usually present and are often normal, but can be of low amplitude or immature. Auditory brainstem evoked responses tend to be normal and do not appear to be a good marker for the development of cerebral palsy. It is also of interest that head growth can be normal in children who develop cerebral palsy. The apparent change in growth coincided with a fall in the rate of length and weight gain.

On clinical examination the children are often extremely irritable up to six months of age, when they tend to become more sociable. The trunk control can be good during the first year, but often deteriorates subsequently. Spasticity of the limbs is usually not very apparent before five to six months of age, but then increases rapidly. All children with these lesions develop a squint, although many have good vision.

In the following three cases periventricular leukomalacia was not diagnosed during the early neonatal period.

Case 13

Premature infant born at 30 weeks gestation. He had a cardio–pulmonary arrest during a lumbar puncture at eight weeks of age. Ultrasound examination at that time revealed cystic periventricular leukomalacia. Subsequently he developed spastic diplegia with a normal intellect.

Ultrasound: An ultrasound during the first week of life was normal and no further scans were performed. On admission to our unit after the cardio–pulmonary arrest at 38 weeks postmenstrual age, a few periventricular cystic lesions were seen (**143**) (arrow), and at six months of age there was mild ventricular dilatation (**144**).

143

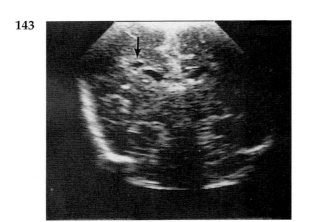

144

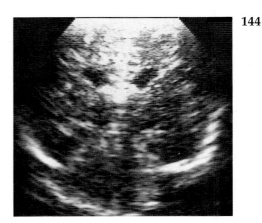

145

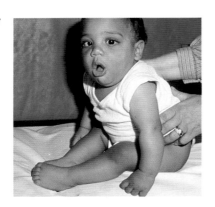

146

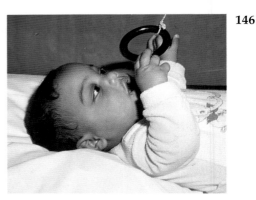

147

Clinical examination: At 38 weeks PMA he was very irritable and had abnormal finger posturing (**145**). At six months he was more sociable and could reach out and grasp a dangling ring (**146**). He sat with some support (**147**) and had a pronounced squint.

Marked tiptoeing was present when he was held in a standing position (**148**). At 30 months he could not stand without support (**149**) but he showed good hand manipulation. An alternating strabismus was present (**150**).

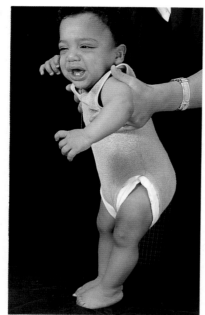

148

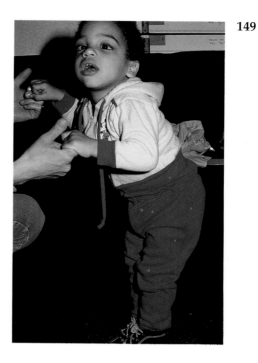

149

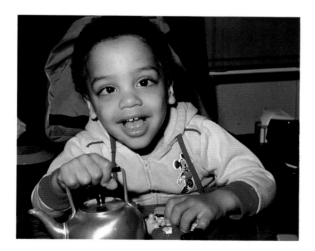

150

Magnetic Resonance Imaging: At five months bilateral areas of low signal intensity were seen at the level of the centrum semiovale (**151**). The inversion recovery scan at the mid-ventricular level showed mildly dilated and irregular ventricles, especially posteriorly. Very little white matter was seen and low signal intensity areas (dark) were seen in the periventricular regions (**152**). There was no change in the ventricles at 18 months but there had been an increase in myelination especially posteriorly (**153**).

151

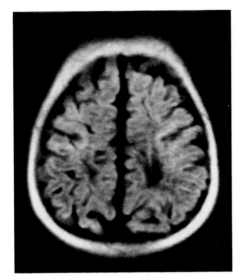

152

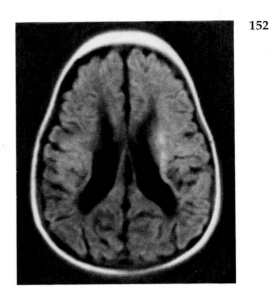

153

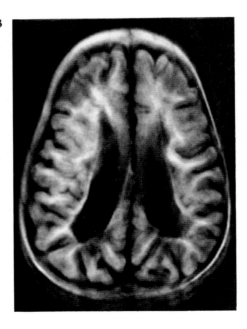

At the level of the centrum semiovale the inversion recovery image showed myelination and prominent sulci (**154**). The short TI inversion recovery scan showed lesions of high signal intensity in both hemispheres (**155**) which were difficult to identify in **154**.

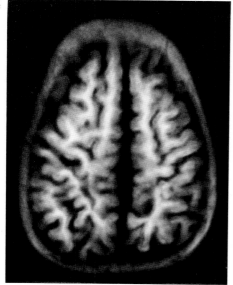
154

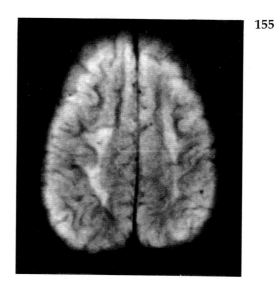
155

Comment: If this infant had not been scanned at 38 weeks, his later problems would have been attributed to his collapse at that time. Although cysts were still present on admission, they were seen only in the fronto–parietal region. Magnetic resonance imaging studies showed irregular occipital horns suggestive of earlier occipital involvement. Note the similarity in MRI appearances between this child and the previous case (case 12). The later severity of the disease was another similarity, although there were some differences in clinical signs.

Clinical examination on admission also supported the diagnosis of cystic periventricular leukomalacia, with the characteristic irritability and finger posturing.

In the following two cases (14 and 15), the diagnosis of cerebral palsy was made on clinical examination after six months of age, and periventricular leukomalacia was confirmed with magnetic resonance imaging.

Case 14

Premature infant, one of twins, born at 30 weeks gestation. He required head box oxygen for a few days and was referred back to the local hospital at the end of his first week. No ultrasound abnormalities other than a small germinal layer haemorrhage were reported at this time. He had obvious signs of spastic diplegia at nine months of age.

Ultrasound: The video recording of his ultrasound scans during the first week of life was reviewed when the diagnosis of cerebral palsy was made. Areas of increased echogenicity (upper arrows) and a right-sided germinal layer haemorrhage (lower arrow) were seen (**156**). After transfer back to the local hospital no further scans were performed.

Clinical examination: At 15 months of age he showed marked scissoring of the legs (**157**). His hand manipulation was good and his eye–hand

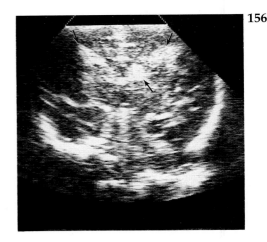

156

coordination and performance were normal for his age (**158**). At four years he was able to walk a few steps using crutches (**159**).

157

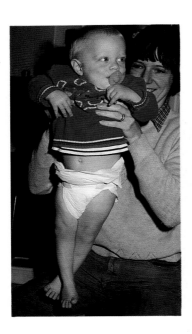

158

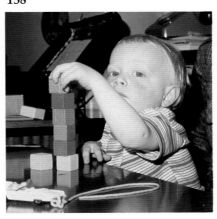

159

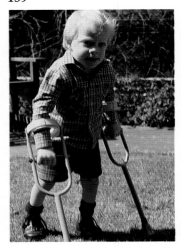

Magnetic Resonance Imaging: Inversion recovery scans were obtained on the child and his twin brother at 18 and 33 months of age. At the midventricular level at 18 months the posterior horns of the lateral ventricles were irregular (**161**). Although the same tracts were myelinated in both children, the myelin was finer in the affected twin (compare **160** and **161**). At age 33 months, at the level of the centrum semiovale, the difference in myelination between the normal (**162**) and the affected (**163**) brother was more obvious. Low signal intensity areas were seen (arrows) within white matter in the affected twin (**163**).

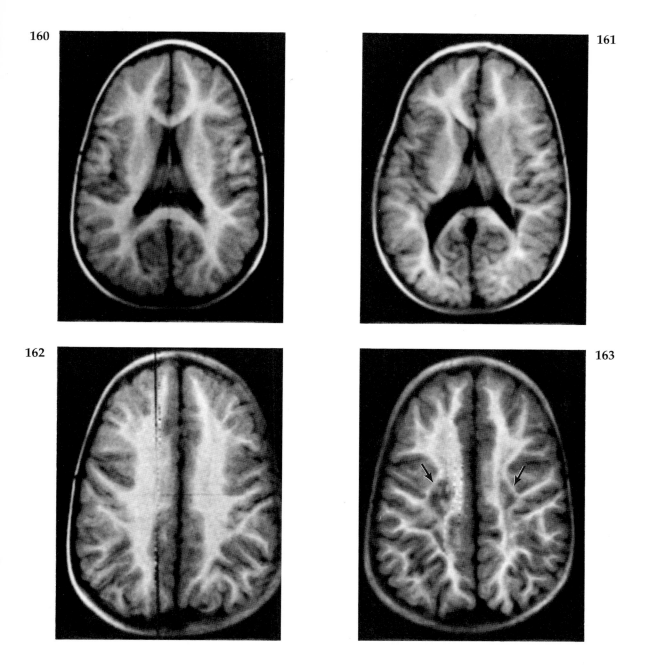

160

161

162

163

Comment: In this case we were able to diagnose retrospectively the early echogenic phase of leukomalacia since a video recording of the early ultrasound scans was available. MRI studies done later during infancy would suggest that these densities subsequently evolved into cystic lesions.

Periventricular densities are quite common, and most are transient and do not evolve into extensive cystic lesions. However, unless children are scanned on a regular basis, for several weeks, extensive cystic lesions can easily be missed. Unfortunately, relatively well infants may be discharged early from the intensive care unit and ultrasound equipment will not always be available in the local hospital.

Case 15

Female infant, born at full term by emergency cae-sarean section following an antepartum haemor-rhage. Her development was considered normal until four months of age. She later developed spastic diplegia, but had a normal intellect.

She was referred to us at two and a half years of age. The diagnosis of spastic diplegia was made on clinical examination, and the presence of leukoma-lacia was confirmed with magnetic resonance imaging.

No **ultrasound** studies were done in the neona-tal period.

Clinical examination: There was increased ex-tensor tone in her legs, with a tendency to scissor, and spontaneous Babinski response on the right (**164**). Her lateral tilting reactions were absent (**165**) but she was able to sit unsupported for a short time (**166**).

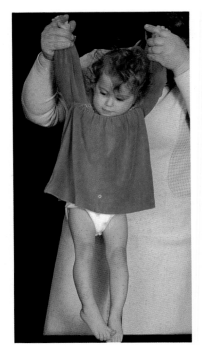

164

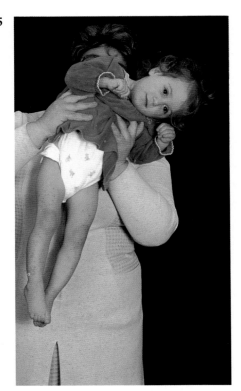

165

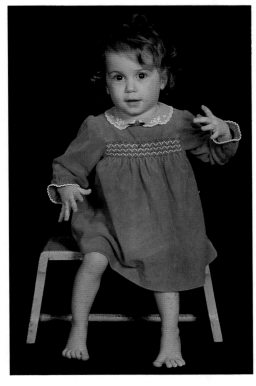

166

Magnetic Resonance Imaging: She was scanned when aged two and half years. The inversion recovery scan through the centrum semiovale showed areas of low signal intensity (dark) within white matter posteriorly (arrows) (**167**). These lesions were highlighted on the short TI inversion recovery sequence (arrows) (**168**). At a low ventricular level the occipital horns were irregular and there was a mild delay in myelin posteriorly (**169**). The short TI inversion recovery scan showed high signal intensity posteriorly (**170**).

Comment: Irregular occipital horns and high signal intensity on the short TI inversion recovery images were present in all of our cases of periventricular cystic leukomalacia which developed spastic diplegia. Although no early ultrasound scans were available in this infant, it was possible to make a retrospective diagnosis of leukomalacia with the use of MRI. An antepartum haemorrhage is known to increase the risk for the development of periventricular leukomalacia, and it is likely that this condition occurred either antenatally or in the immediate perinatal period.

Mixed leukomalacia

Case 16

Premature infant, the first of twins, born at 34 weeks gestation by an emergency caesarean section following cord prolapse. She was well initially, but deteriorated suddenly on day 11, with necrotising enterocolitis. She developed mixed cystic leukomalacia, and at three years of age she was quadriplegic, microcephalic, cortically blind and severely mentally retarded.

Ultrasound: None was available before her referral to our unit on day 15 when she perforated her gut, complicating the course of necrotising enterocolitis. At that time, areas of increased echogenicity were seen around the anterior horns of the ventricles (**171**). Extensive cystic lesions developed in the echogenic areas. The parasagittal view showed the cystic lesions extending deep into the white matter (**172**). The cysts were seen up to six months, when the anterior fontanelle closed.

A **CT** scan at six weeks of age showed extensive areas of decreased attenuation in both hemispheres (**173**). At eight months of age, cystic lesions were visible adjacent to the mildly dilated ventricles (**174**).

171

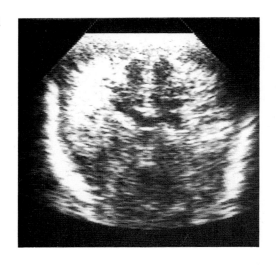

172

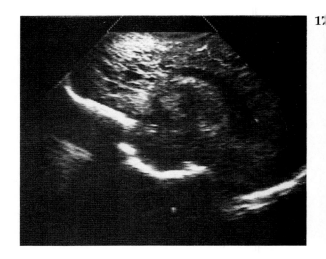

173

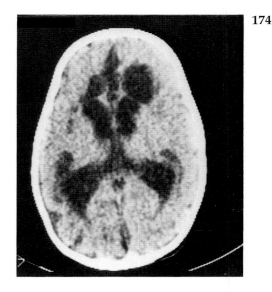

174

No consistent **visual evoked responses** could be elicited at 40 weeks postmenstrual age, but the child showed an excellent tracking response (**175**).

Clinical examination at nine months showed definite signs of cerebral palsy, and the child had lost her ability to track. There was a marked tendency for her to jackknife backwards when held in a sitting position (**176**). At 15 months there was a marked delay in development compared with her unaffected twin (**177**).

175

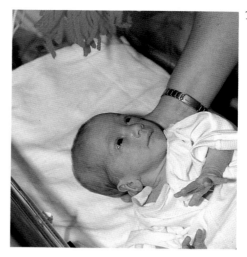

176

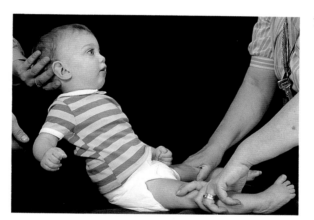

177

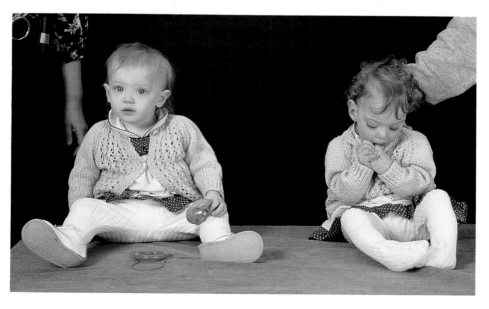

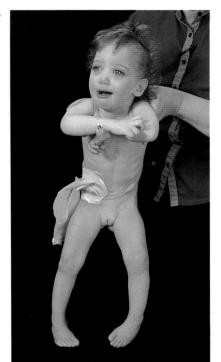

At 18 months of age she showed an abnormal posture and increased extensor tone when held in a standing position (**178**), and she was unable to sit without support (**179**).

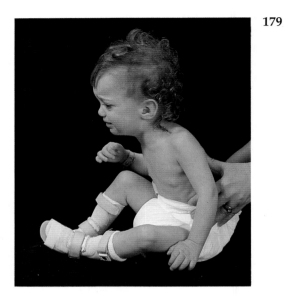

The head circumference chart showed growth parallel to, but below, the 10th centile up to seven months of age, corrected for prematurity. From seven months there was no further growth (**180**).

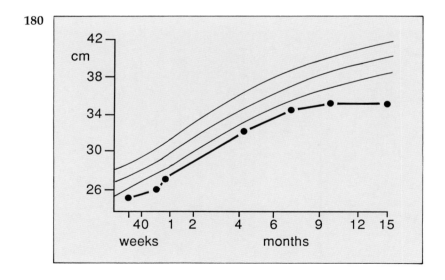

Magnetic Resonance Imaging: Inversion recovery scans are shown at 21 and 33 months of age. A comparison between the twin sisters at 21 months showed a marked difference in the degree of myelination (**181** and **182**). Myelinated white matter was seen only in the thalami in the affected twin (**182**). The ventricles were dilated and extensive areas of low signal intensity were seen in the periventricular regions.

181

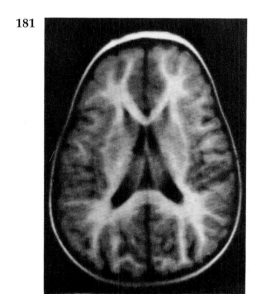

182

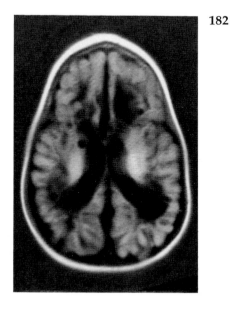

183

A repeat inversion recovery scan at 33 months showed little progression in myelination (**183**).

Comment: This case illustrates a severe form of mixed cystic leukomalacia. She became cortically blind during the first year of her life. It is of interest that, clinically, vision was normal in the infants under study until about 48–52 weeks postmenstrual age, and the visual deficit did not necessarily correlate with occipital involvement. Cysts were much more prominent anteriorly. The progress of myelination was extremely poor in this child with mixed leukomalacia, compared to the children with periventricular leukomalacia. This case is similar to case 6 (in the postmortem series), where only fine strands of myelin were seen extending towards the cortex at the same age.

Case 17

Premature infant born at 28 weeks gestation with mild respiratory distress syndrome. He required ventilation for the first 48 hours. A severe deterioration in his clinical condition occurred at two weeks of age, when he developed necrotising enterocolitis. Initially he was treated conservatively, but underwent surgery for a stricture at seven weeks of age.

On admission he had marked abdominal distension and was lying in an extended posture (184).

Electroencephalogram: Continuous 4-channel EEG recorded following admission showed excessive discontinuity and low amplitude (185).

Ultrasound: During the first week of life the scans were reported as normal, and no scans were done following the development of necrotising enterocolitis. At 35 weeks postmenstrual age he had established cystic leukomalacia. The cysts extended deep into the white matter from the lateral ventricles, especially on the left (186) (arrow). In the parasagittal view, the cystic areas were localised in the parietal region (187) (arrow). At four months the cysts could not be identified, but moderate ventricular dilatation and marked widening of the interhemispheric fissure were present (188).

184

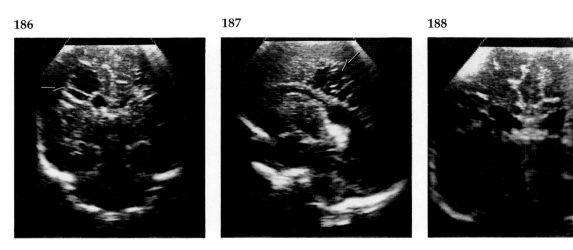

185

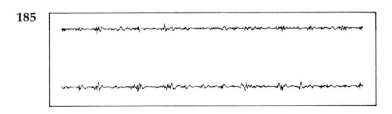

186   **187**   **188**

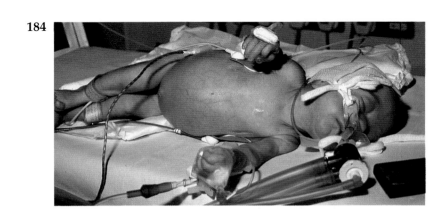

Visual Evoked Responses performed at 40 weeks postmenstrual age were of low voltage, but a positivity followed by a negativity was present (**189**).

Clinical examination: At 40 weeks postmenstrual age he was extremely irritable. Frequent spontaneous startles and tremors were observed (**190**) and the thumbs were adducted. At four months of age he was still extremely irritable and there was marked tightness of the popliteal angles (**191**). At this age he could not focus or follow, and cortical blindness was suspected.

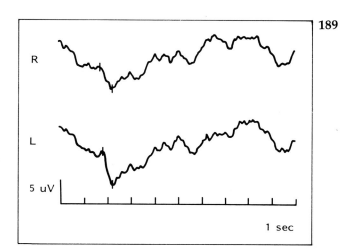

189

R

L

5 uV

1 sec

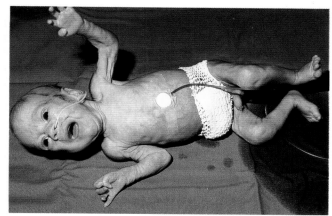

190

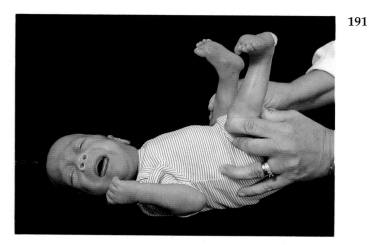

191

At 16 months he was still unable to lift his head when prone (192). His visual function was still extremely poor, but had improved slightly. At two years he was more responsive and his visual function had improved further. When prone, he was able to lift his head and chest off the floor for a short period (193), but he required considerable support to sit (194).

192

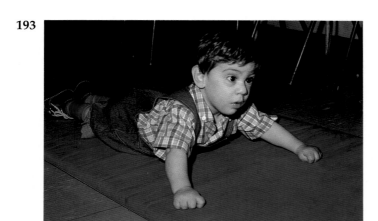

193

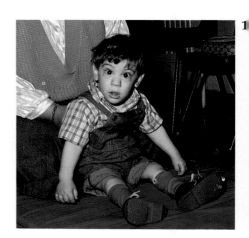

Magnetic Resonance Imaging: The inversion recovery sequence at 13 months showed moderately dilated and irregular ventricles, with a small porencephalic cyst on the right (arrow), and very little white matter was seen (195). There were focal areas of low signal intensity throughout both hemispheres. At 24 months (196) the inversion recovery sequence showed little change in the ventricular contour, but there was some progress in myelination anteriorly and laterally. At the low ventricular level at the same age the posterior horns were slightly dilated, and myelination was markedly delayed (197). Areas of high signal intensity were seen in the periventricular regions, extending towards the cortex anteriorly on the short TI inversion recovery sequence (198).

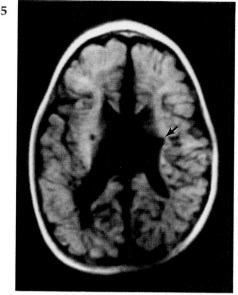

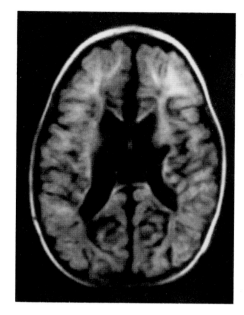

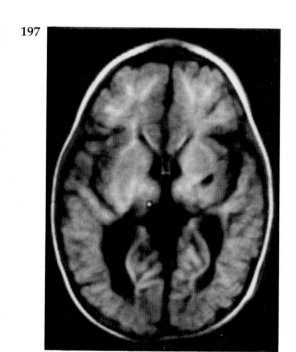

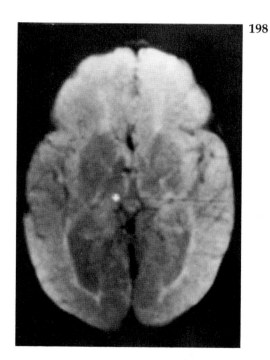

Comment: This infant showed a relatively mild course of mixed cystic leukomalacia. Infants with lesions extending towards the subcortical areas are much more likely to present with cortical blindness and mental retardation later in infancy. In this infant there appeared to be a loss of vision around five months of age, but later recovery occurred. Infants with these lesions also show signs of a quadriplegia, with more arm than leg involvement. The progress of myelination is poor compared to infants with only periventricular lesions, but in both infants with extensive mixed leukomalacia some progress in myelination was seen.

Subcortical leukomalacia

Case 18

Premature infant born at 30 weeks gestation. An antenatal diagnosis of gastroschizis was made and surgery was performed shortly after delivery (199). She made an uneventful recovery and at three weeks of age was transferred back to her local hospital. Ten days later she was re-admitted with necrotising enterocolitis and gram negative septicaemia. She developed subcortical leukomalacia and became quadriplegic, cortically blind and severely mentally retarded.

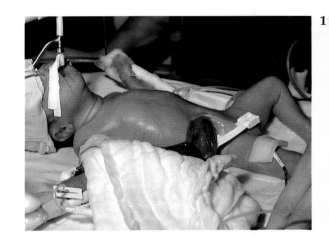

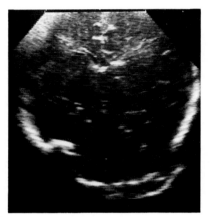

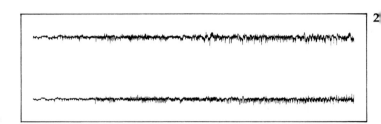

Ultrasound: A coronal view during the first week was normal (200). Areas of increased echogenicity were only seen six days following the onset of necrotising enterocolitis. However, a continuous four-channel **EEG** was very abnormal, with seizures on a low amplitude background on the day of her second admission (201).

The areas of increased echogenicity were most marked around the interhemispheric fissure and above the corpus callosum in the sagittal midline view (202).

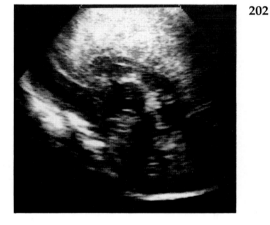

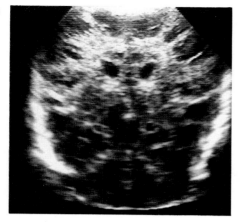

203

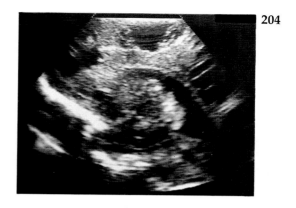

204

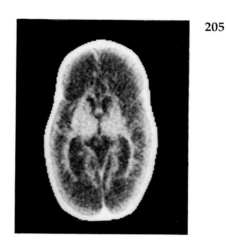

205

Ten days later these areas broke down into large cystic areas in subcortical white matter (**203** and **204**).

A **CT** scan at this stage showed extensive areas of decreased attenuation throughout both hemispheres (**205**).

Auditory Brainstem Evoked Responses at 36 and 40 weeks postmenstrual age showed an abnormal V:I ratio at 60 dB intensity, due to an abnormally low amplitude of wave V (**206**).

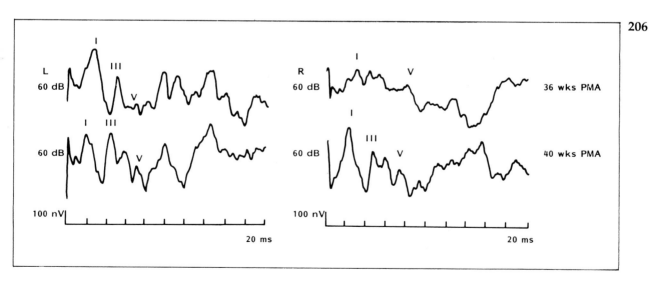

206

Clinical examination: At 40 weeks postmenstrual age she showed many abnormal signs, including extreme irritability, marked arm flexion and leg extension, a persistently flexed left forefinger (**207**) and extension of the big toes. Once she settled it was possible to get an excellent tracking response (**208**), but at six months of age she was no longer able to follow. Her head circumference was far below the third centile (**209**), while her weight and length were on the 25th centile.

207

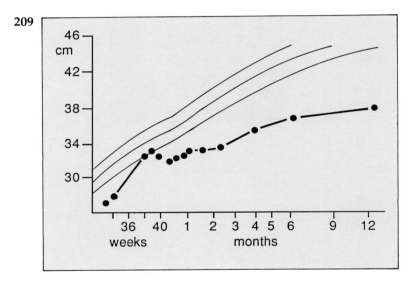

209

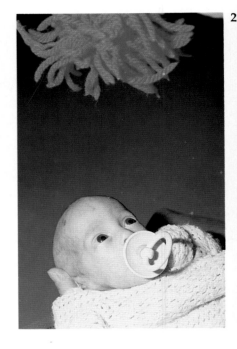

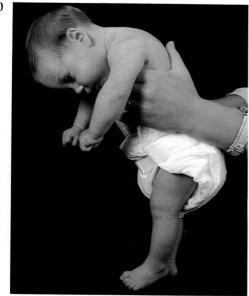

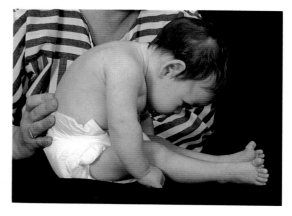

At six months her limb tone was increased, more so in the arms than in the legs. Poor trunk control was displayed when she was held in a standing (**210**) or sitting position (**211**). An increased extensor tone was seen in her limbs and she had spontaneous extension of her big toes. At eight months of age the absence of trunk control was well shown in ventral suspension (**212**). By 18 months, little progress was seen; she was still unable to sit unsupported (**213**), and had increased extensor tone when held in the standing position (**214**).

212

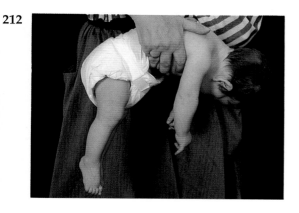

214

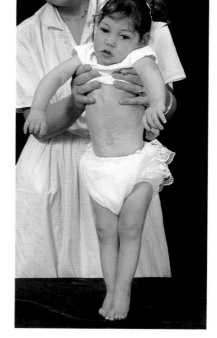

213

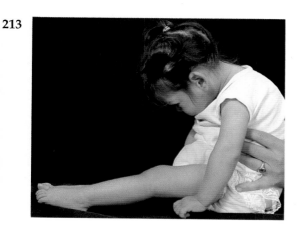

A spontaneous asymmetrical tonic neck reflex was present (**215**) and there was marked tightness of her popliteal angles (**216**).

215

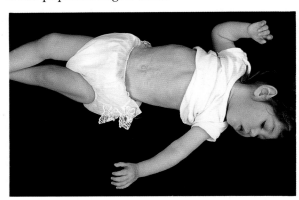

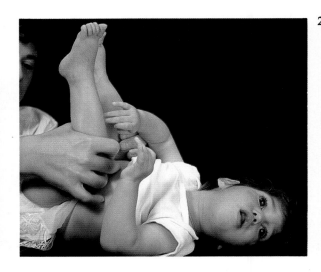

Magnetic Resonance Imaging: The inversion recovery scan at four months showed an increased subarachnoid space and ventricular dilatation. Extensive low signal intensity areas were also present within both hemispheres (**217**). By 12 months there had been an increase in brain size with an increase in the size of the ventricles and a decrease in the subarachnoid space (**218**). No myelin was seen in this child above the tentorium.

217

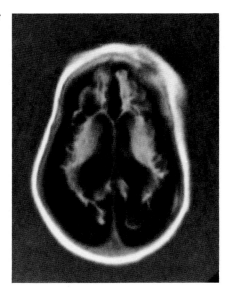

218

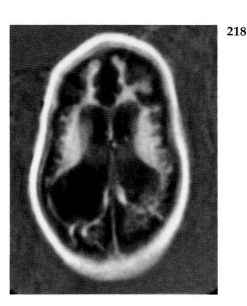

Comment: This case illustrates that leukomalacia can occur much later in the neonatal period following a severe insult. The distribution of the lesions relates more to the time of the insult than the gestational age at birth. Hence, in this infant born at 30 weeks gestation, the deterioration occurred at 34 weeks and her lesions were predominantly in the subcortical regions. She also illustrates the typical clinical picture at 40 weeks postmenstrual age, which is similar in infants with both periventricular and subcortical lesions. However, whilst infants with periventricular lesions may show some improvement by six months of age, those with subcortical leukomalacia show definite signs of quadriplegia and cortical blindness at this age.

Case 19

Premature infant born at 33 weeks gestation. She suffered severe birth asphyxia following an abruptio placentae. She developed severe quadriplegia, cortical blindness, and severe mental retardation.

Electroencephalogram: Continuous 4-channel EEG recorded on day 2 showed an isoelectric recording (**219**).

Ultrasound: On day 3 the brain had a 'fuzzy' appearance in the coronal plane (**220**). The anatomical structures were difficult to define and pulsations were practically absent. Her intracranial pressure was measured following insertion of a subarachnoid catheter, and was markedly raised (33mmHg, normal <6mmHg). Her cerebral perfusion pressure was very low (<10, normal >30mmHg), and several doses of Mannitol were given over a 24-hour period. Areas of increased echogenicity were seen on day 7 and the lateral ventricles were slightly dilated (**221**). Subcortical cystic leukomalacia developed and the subcortical cysts were still present at seven months (**222**).

219

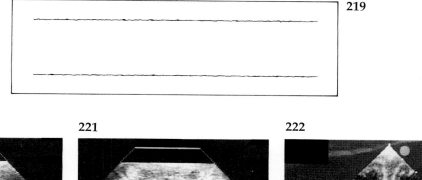

220

221

222

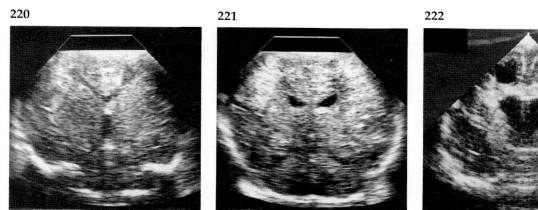

A **CT** scan at 11 days of age showed bilateral thalamic and subarachnoid haemorrhages (**223**), which were not seen on ultrasound.

At four weeks of age, extensive areas of decreased attenuation were visible throughout both hemispheres (**224**).

223

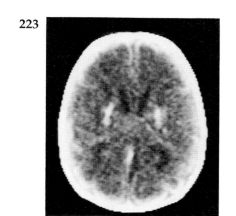

224

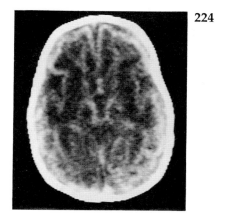

125

225

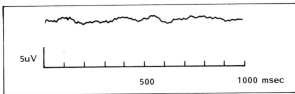

5uV

500   1000 msec

226

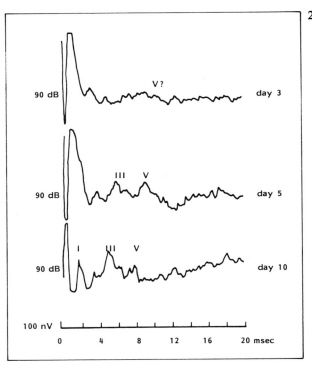

90 dB   V ?   day 3

90 dB   III   V   day 5

90 dB   I   III   V   day 10

100 nV

0   4   8   12   16   20 msec

Visual Evoked Responses: at 37 weeks post-menstrual age no responses could be elicited (**225**).

Auditory Brainstem Evoked Responses were done on days 3, 5 and 10 at 90 dB intensity; the waves were difficult to identify on day 3 (**226**), but wave V was probably present. Recovery occurred during the next week, and waves I, III and V were clearly seen on day 10, although the I:V ratio was abnormal.

At 40 weeks postmenstrual age the **EEG** was still abnormal, with excessive discontinuity, low amplitude and seizure activity (**227**).

227

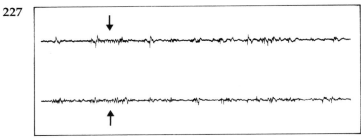

Clinical examination: At 38 weeks postmenstrual age she showed marked extension of her legs and partial flexion of her left arm (**228**) and her posture was abnormal for an infant of this gestation. At six months her development was better than anticipated, and she was able to sit with some support (**229**).

228

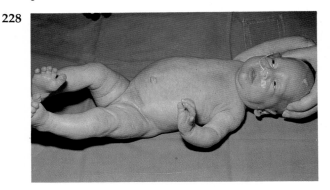

229

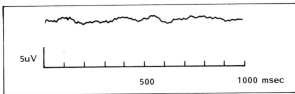

Her head circumference, however, was below the 3rd centile (230). She had abnormal 'stretching' movements of her arms (231), and movements suggestive of infantile spasms. Hypsarrythmia was diagnosed on the electroencephalogram. At two years she was overtly retarded and cortically blind. She was still unable to sit unsupported (232). She was quadriplegic, but extremely hypotonic (233).

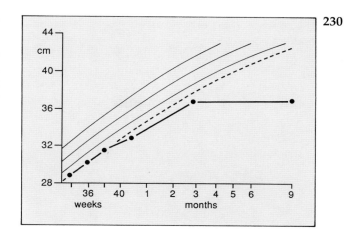

230

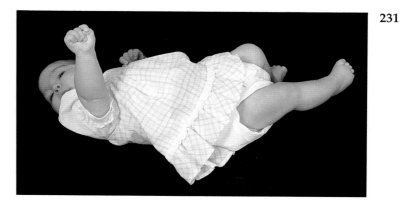

231

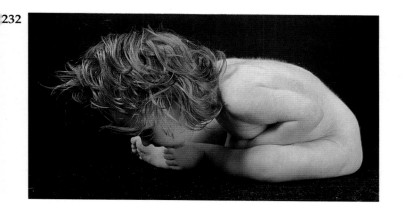

232

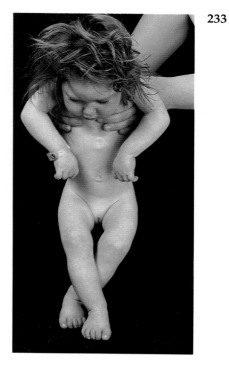

233

Magnetic Resonance Imaging: the inversion recovery sequences at 35 weeks showed extensive areas of low signal intensity throughout both hemispheres in the centrum semiovale (**234**), and the subarachnoid space was increased. At five months there had been some shrinkage of the areas of low signal intensity, but there was marked cortical atrophy and no myelin was visible (**235**). At 24 months there were still extensive areas of low signal intensity in both hemispheres (**236**), and no myelin was present above the tentorium.

234

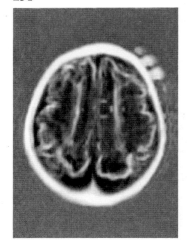

235

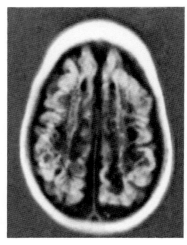

236

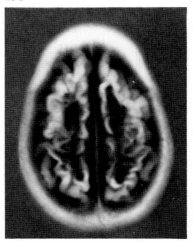

Comment: This case illustrates the fact that thalamic haemorrhages may be missed with ultrasonography. The CT scan may give additional information in this early stage, but during the cystic phase US is superior to CT. In contrast to the periventricular cystic lesions, which tend to disappear after 2–4 months, subcortical cysts are seen with ultrasound until the fontanelle closes.

Her auditory brainstem evoked responses were almost absent when her EEG was isoelectric, but a good recovery of the ABR was seen within a week. An abnormal wave V:I ratio was still present at this stage. This finding has been noted in both cases of subcortical leukomalacia and has been reported as a useful marker for a poor outcome.

A comparison of all our survivors with extensive cystic leukomalacia stresses the importance, not only of making the diagnosis of extensive cystic leukomalacia, but also of looking at the distribution of the cystic lesions. The site and size of these lesions provide an excellent marker for later prognosis.

Relatively small anterior lesions appear to be associated with transient dystonia. When the lesions are more extensive, permanent motor signs are present. Spasticity, however, is much less a dominant feature. Poor muscle control and balance predominate. The more the lesions extend into the frontal subcortical areas, the more likelihood there is for mental retardation and probably infantile spasms. Surprisingly, the periventricular lesions in the occipital areas are not usually associated with visual deficits but are markers for

marked spasticity involving the legs more than the arms. With extension into the subcortical areas, either anteriorly or posteriorly, the arms become more involved, and mental retardation and cortical blindness are common.

Figure **237** summarises the clinical differences between children with extensive cystic periventricular and subcortical leukomalacias.

Electrophysiological changes, too, show differences. In the periventricular cystic leukomalacias, abnormalities, though present, are transient, whereas with subcortical lesions tend to be persistent.

There are also marked differences in the progress in myelination depending on the size of the lesion. Good progress can be seen with the periventricular lesions, and complete absence of myelination may occur with the subcortical lesion.

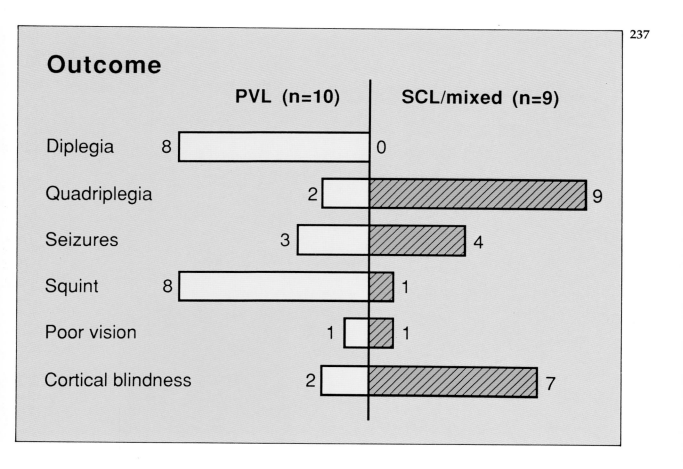

237

A comparison of Intraventricular Haemorrhage and Periventricular Leukomalacia

The final two cases in this chapter illustrate premature twins, one with leukomalacia, the other with haemorrhage.

Cases 20/21
Premature infants born at 27 weeks gestation. The girl developed an intraventricular haemorrhage (arrow) (**238**), and the boy cystic periventricular leukomalacia (**239**).

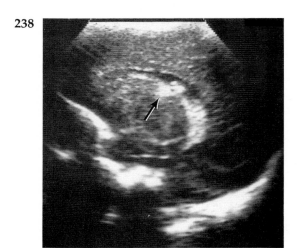

238

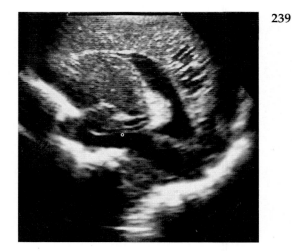

239

Clinical examination at 38 weeks postmenstrual age showed a marked difference between the two infants. In the supine position, the girl showed flexion of her legs (**240**), while the boy had extended posture of his legs and a flexed arm posture (**241**).

In ventral suspension, the trunk tone was slightly decreased in the girl (**242**), but increased in the boy (**243**). There was no tightness of the popliteal angles in the girl (**244**), but there was marked tightness in the boy (**245**).

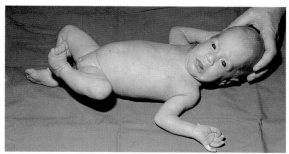

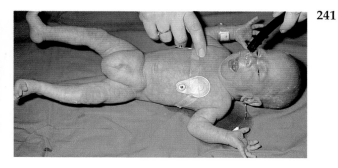

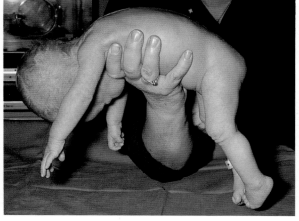

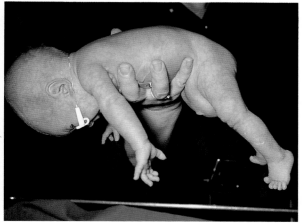

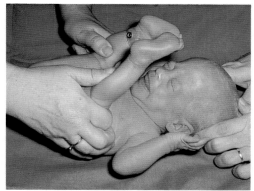

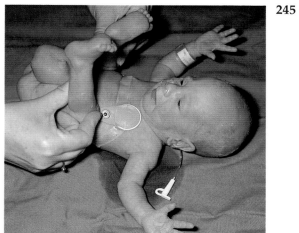

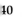

When reassessed at seven months the girl could almost sit without support and reached out for an object (246), whereas the boy could not sit unsupported (247). In ventral suspension the girl had her head above the plane of her body and showed leg elevation (248), but the boy kept his head below the plane of his body and had an extended leg posture (249). There were marked differences in the popliteal angles – greater than 140° in the girl (250) and less than 100° in the boy (251). The girl had full abduction of her hips (252), but this was markedly reduced in the boy (253). Standing, the girl danced (254), but the boy showed increased extensor tone (255).

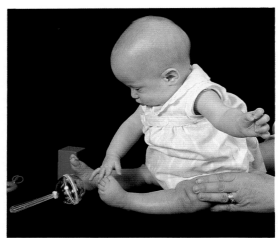

246

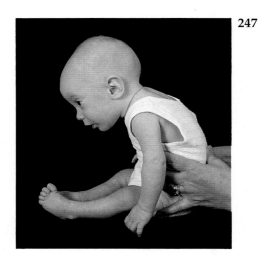

247

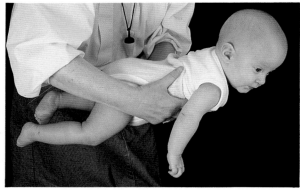

248

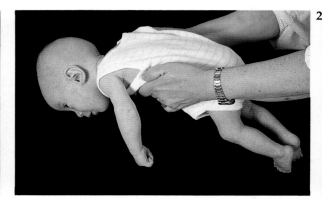

2

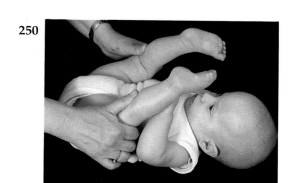
250

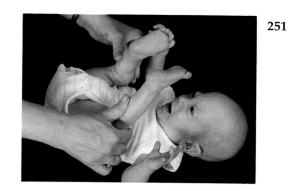
251

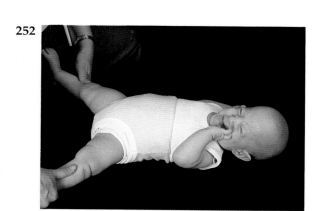
252

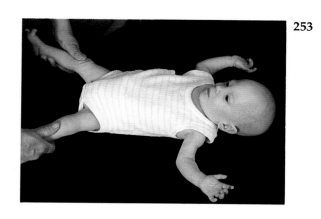
253

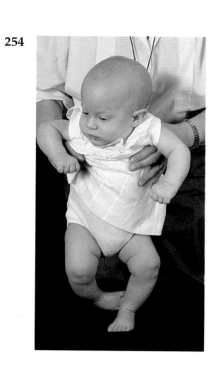
254

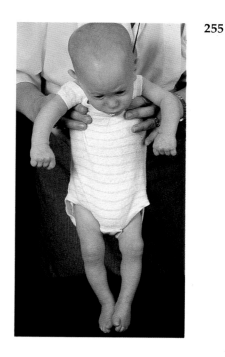
255

Magnetic Resonance Imaging: The boy was examined at 12 months and showed the typical features of periventricular leukomalacia. The inversion recovery sequence at the mid-ventricular level showed slightly dilated ventricles with irregular and sharply angled occipital horns. Myelination was delayed, especially posteriorly (**256**). Myelin was seen at the level of the centrum semiovale (**257**), and high signal intensity areas were seen on the short TI inversion recovery sequence (**258**).

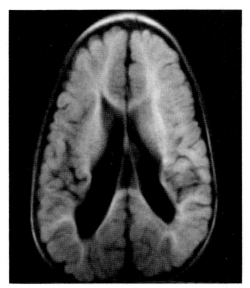

256

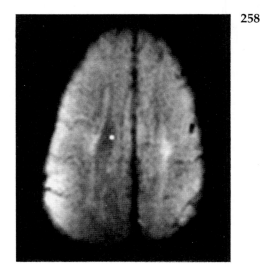

257

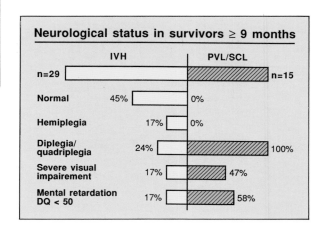

258

Comment: These twin infants showed typical patterns of development: hypotonia, which resolved during the first year of life in a child with an intraventricular haemorrhage; and spastic diplegia in a child with cystic periventricular leukomalacia. The difference was already obvious during the neonatal period.

Only a few of our premature infants who survived with a large intraventricular or parenchymal haemorrhage have been discussed in this chapter. 45% of all our survivors with this type of lesion did not develop any major neurological abnormalities and only 17% had severe handicap with mental retardation (DQ<70, uncorrected for prematurity).

Neurological status in survivors ≥ 9 months

	IVH	PVL/SCL
	n=29	n=15
Normal	45%	0%
Hemiplegia	17%	0%
Diplegia/ quadriplegia	24%	100%
Severe visual impairement	17%	47%
Mental retardation DQ < 50	17%	58%

Chapter 4. Cerebral Artery Infarction

Historical Background

Friede (1875) described five cases of cerebral artery infarction and reviewed the earlier pathological literature. Barmada *et al* (1979) defined the lesion as a severe disorganisation or even complete disruption of grey and white matter, caused by embolic, thrombotic or ischaemic events.

Pathological Features

Cerebral artery infarction – 'neonatal stroke' – is more commonly seen in full term infants, but has also been noted in premature infants. The lesion is 3–4 times more common in the left hemisphere, and infarction of the middle cerebral artery occurs with twice the frequency of that of other arteries. In the acute stage, the hemisphere is swollen and deeply congested. Involvement of both white matter and cortex is seen in secondary haemorrhagic infarction in some cases. In those who survive for a longer period, contraction of the affected area is observed, with softening and multicystic degeneration, giving a honeycomb appearance on sectioning. Large porencephalic cysts can also be found in some cases.

Clinical Recognition

It is possible to make the diagnosis using **Ultrasound**, but additional imaging studies are required. It is not possible to distinguish between haemorrhagic and non-haemorrhagic lesions using ultrasound alone. The timing of an **X-ray Computed Tomographic (CT)** examination is important. If possible it should be done at one week following the onset of the lesion. On a CT within 48 hours the lesion may be missed, and after more than one week the blood may be isodense and not visible. Using the appropriate pulse sequence it is possible to differentiate between haemorrhagic and non-haemorrhagic infarction with MRI.

Clinical examination: Term infants with infarction usually present with clinical unilateral seizures. Asymmetry in tone is usually found and tends to persist. Seizures are uncommon in premature infants. Hypotonia and asymmetry can be seen at 40 weeks postmenstrual age.

Electrophysiological Tests

Auditory Brainstem Evoked Responses and **Visual Evoked Responses** were not abnormal or asymmetrical in our limited number of infants. However, an asymmetry in the VER might be expected in infants with infarcts of the posterior cerebral artery.

Electroencephalogram (EEG) can be very useful, especially in term infants who usually present with clinical seizures. In preterm infants, asymmetries with unilateral sharp waves can be found, but usually on a normal background activity.

Case Histories

Case 1

Premature infant born at 33 weeks gestation, the first of twins. He was well until day 3, when he developed a gram negative septicaemia and disseminated intravascular coagulopathy. A localised infarct was diagnosed. He showed a transient asymmetry in tone during the first year of life. The asymmetry persisted but improved, and he was able to walk at 19 months.

Ultrasound: The scans were normal during the first three days. Following a clinical deterioration, a wedge-shaped echogenic area was seen on the right side in the coronal view with the scan head angled backwards (**1**), and in the parasagittal view (**2**).

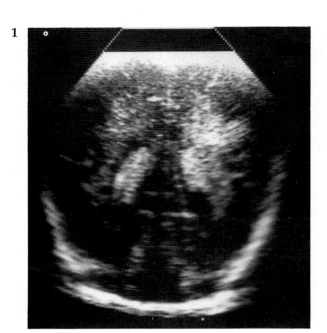
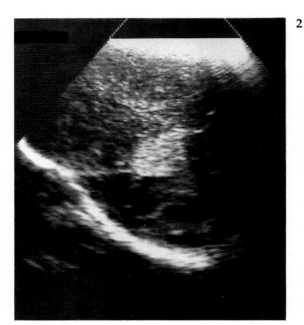

Electroencephalogram: Continuous 4-channel EEG at this time showed right-sided sharp waves (arrow) but no seizure activity (**3**).

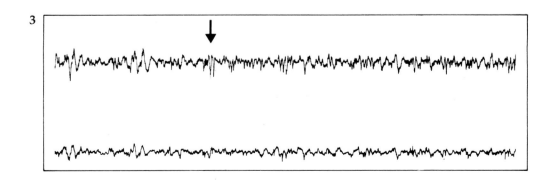

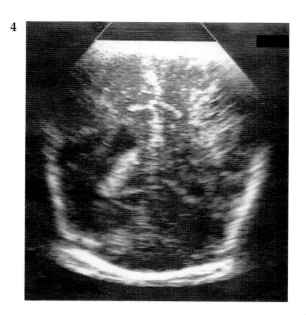

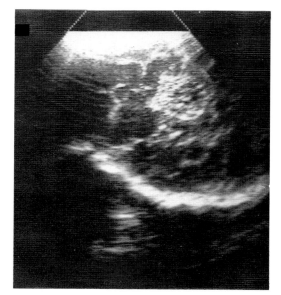

The echogenic areas broke down into small, honeycomb-like cysts in both coronal and sagittal views (**4** and **5**).

CT: The scan on day 9 was within normal limits. (**6**).

Magnetic Resonance Imaging: An inversion recovery sequence at 37 weeks postmenstrual age is shown. There was a wedge-shaped area of low signal intensity in the right parieto–temporal region (arrows) (**7**). There was no evidence of a haemorrhage on this image, although this was suggested by the ultrasound findings.

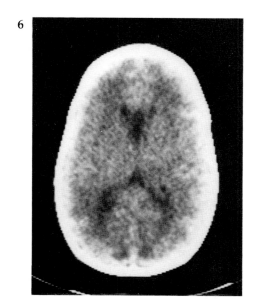

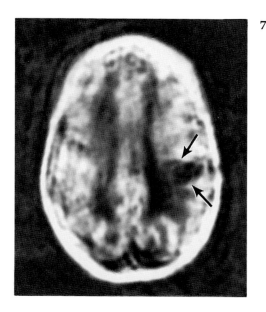

Clinical examination: At six months he showed some asymmetry of tone. The thumb was adducted on both sides (**8**), and there was a difference in the popliteal angles (**9**). At nine months of age the asymmetry was less marked (**10**) and he was able to sit with slight support (**11**).

8
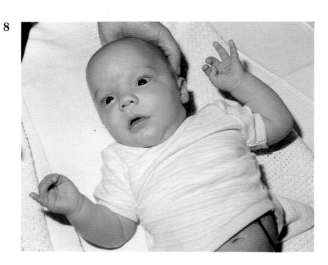

9
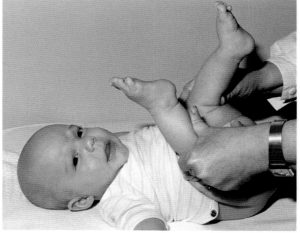

10
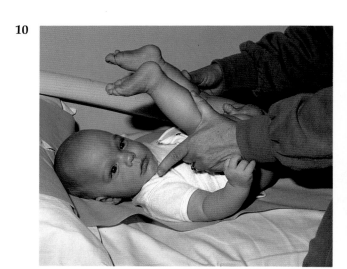

11
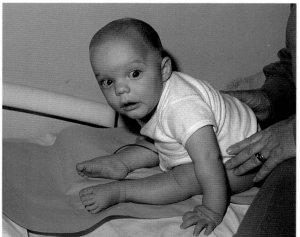

Magnetic Resonance Imaging: At 10 months of age the area of low signal intensity persisted on the inversion recovery (arrow) (**12**), and there was less myelination in this area than on the contralateral side. A short TI inversion recovery sequence showed high signal intensity at the site of the infarct (arrow) (**13**) and in the periventricular regions.

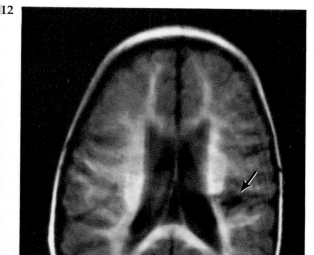

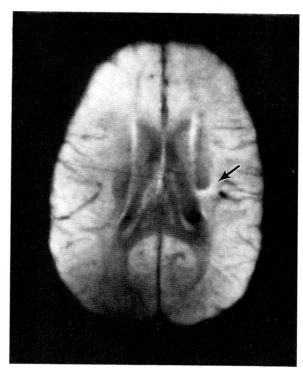

Comment: A differential diagnosis based on the ultrasound examination of this premature infant was either parenchymal haemorrhage or periventricular leukomalacia. However, it would be unusual to see a parenchymal haemorrhage in a premature infant without an associated intraventricular haemorrhage, and periventricular leukomalacia tends to be bilateral rather than unilateral.

The magnetic resonance images supported the diagnosis of a non-haemorrhagic localised infarct, presumably in the distribution of the middle cerebral artery. The lesion was not seen on the CT scan.

In the premature infant, localised infarction is far less common than either a parenchymal haemorrhage or periventricular leukomalacia, but carries a far better prognosis.

Case 2

Premature infant born at 31 weeks gestation with no perinatal problems. A localised infarct was diagnosed on routine ultrasound scanning and the child developed transient asymmetry of tone during her first year.

Ultrasound: The coronal view on day 2 showed a wedge-shaped area of increased echogenicity around the right occipital horn of the lateral ventricle (**14**) (arrow).

CT: On day 8, the scan showed an area of increased attenuation adjacent to the right occipital horn, indicating the presence of haemorrhage within the lesion (**15**).

Sequential parasagittal ultrasound scans showed the evolution of an area of increased echogenicity (**16**) into a cystic area three weeks later (**17**). This cystic lesion was no longer visible at 40 weeks postmenstrual age.

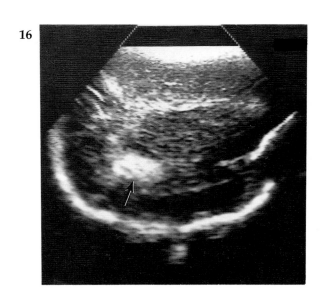

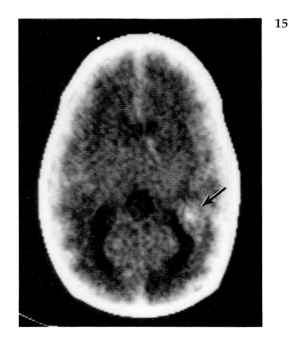

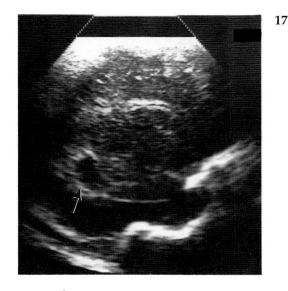

Clinical examination: At two weeks of age there was some asymmetry of tone in her legs, which normalised by the time she was five weeks old. At 15 months she was progressing well (**18**), but was unable to walk independently (**19**). There was no asymmetry of tone.

18

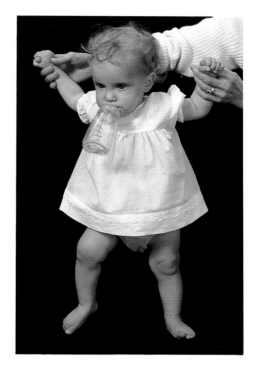

19

20

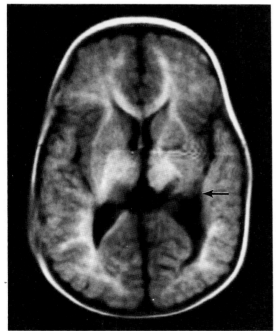

Magnetic Resonance Imaging: At 15 months an inversion recovery scan showed less myelin posteriorly on the right than on the left, and an irregularly shaped right occipital horn (arrow) (**20**).

Comment: By comparing these two premature infants (cases 1 and 2) with localised infarcts and a similar outcome, two interesting points can be made: (i) on the ultrasound scan, the lesions appeared to be differently located on the coronal view, but similar in position on the parasagittal view; (ii) the evolution of the echogenic lesion was different. The child with the non-haemorrhagic lesion developed honeycomb-like cysts, while the haemorrhagic infarct evolved into one cystic lesion.

Case 3

Full term infant born at 39 weeks gestation, following an uncomplicated pregnancy and delivery. Focal right-sided seizures occurred at three hours of age, and a left middle cerebral artery infarction was diagnosed. She developed a right hemiplegia, but had a normal intellect.

Ultrasound on day 1 showed an area of increased echogenicity in the region of the left middle cerebral artery (**21**).

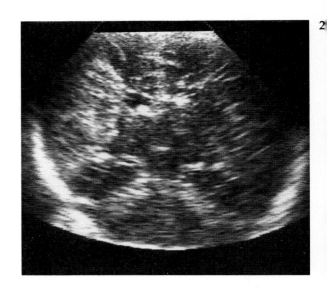

A **CT** scan on day 9 showed areas of high attenuation in the left fronto–temporal region, indicating the presence of a haemorrhagic infarct (**22**).

At two months a porencephalic cyst was seen (**23**), and the left hemisphere was smaller than the right. This cystic lesion could not be identified with ultrasound.

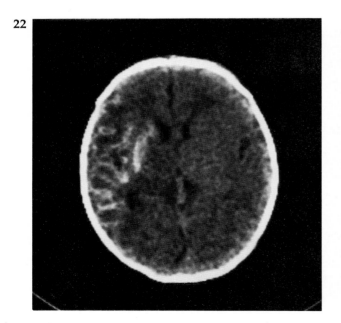

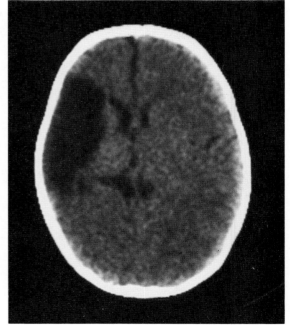

Clinical examination: At 14 months of age she preferred to use her left hand (**24**).

Her right hand was fisted and she only used it occasionally. At two years she walked unaided with a slightly hemiplegic gait. She showed good balance and easily achieved a crouched position (**25**).

24

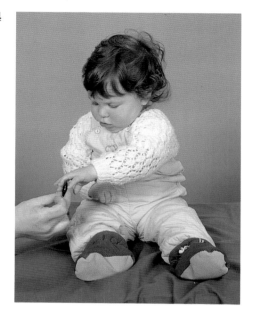

25

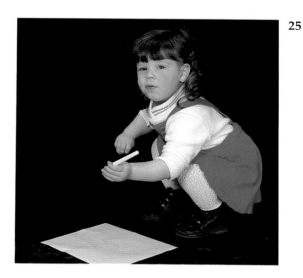

26

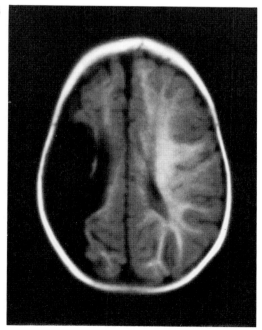

Magnetic Resonance Imaging: The inversion recovery image at 10 months of age showed a large area of low signal intensity in the left hemisphere, with only small amounts of white matter. Myelination was within normal limits in the right hemisphere (**26**).

Comment: This case illustrates the difference in outcome in a term infant with an infarct – often called stroke – and the two previous premature infants (cases 1 and 2).

The term infants tend to develop a marked hemiplegia, while the premature infants are inclined to show transient asymmetry of tone. The difference in outcome between the term and preterm infants might be related to the size of the lesion, which in turn is probably related to the difference in vascular distribution at different ages.

Chapter 5. Haemorrhagic and Ischaemic Lesions of Antenatal Origin

Historical Background

The pathological appearance of haemorrhagic and ischaemic lesions in the foetal brain has been described many times. Larroche (1986) classified their origin in four main groups: maternal, foetal, placental or idiopathic. These groups can be further subdivided as shown below.

Maternal conditions

- Systemic disorders (severe anaemia, severe anoxia, severe pre-eclamptic toxaemia)
- Maternal trauma (direct trauma to maternal abdomen, or shock)
- Gas poisoning (carbon monoxide or butane gas poisoning)
- Maternal coagulopathy (maternal anticoagulants; idiopathic thrombocytopenic purpura)

Foetal Conditions

- Multiple pregnancy (death of one of monozygotic twins)
- Cerebral arterial occlusion (emboli from placental or foetal virus)
- Coagulopathy (isoimmune thrombocytopenia; inherited clotting factor deficiencies)

Complications of Placenta or Cord

- Placental abruption; true knots

Idiopathic

Pathological Features

The appearance of the brain lesions depends on the timing of the intra-uterine insult and the time between the insult and the examination of the brain. Early injury disturbs morphogenesis, while later injuries are more likely to lead to clastic lesions.

Clinical Recognition

Prenatal ultrasound examination is the method of choice for the diagnosis of these conditions. Lesions are sometimes picked up on routine scans during pregnancy; however, on other occasions, ultrasound will be performed because of a maternal history of trauma or a suspicious past history. Several scans may be necessary to identify the lesions. A postnatal scan should be performed as soon as possible to support the antenatal origin of the lesion. **Doppler studies** are also used and will be of help to identify foetuses at risk.

Clinical examination: Interesting data about foetal movements have become available using prenatal ultrasound. Reports of reduced foetal movements or increased repetitive movements (seizures) have been reported following insults to the mother.

Electrophysiological Tests

Cardiotocogram recordings can provide important information about foetal well-being. A cerebral function monitor has also been used antenatally in a few centres.

Case Histories

Case 1

Female infant delivered by an elective caesarean section at 36 weeks gestation. An antenatal ultrasound scan at 34 weeks showed a unilaterally dilated ventricle (**1**)

The child appeared well at birth (**2**), but her ventricular dilatation progressed rapidly. She was shunted at eight weeks and had three shunt revisions during the first year. At four years of age she had a slight asymmetry in tone and some visual impairment.

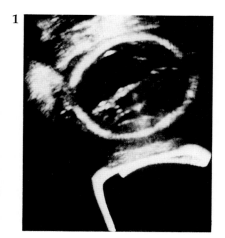

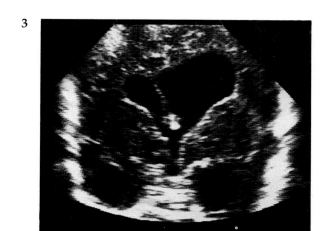

Ultrasound: Immediately after birth her scan confirmed marked dilatation of the right ventricle, with only moderate dilatation of the left ventricle (**3**), suggesting an old intraventricular and parenchymal haemorrhage. At four weeks of age her head circumference exceeded the 90th centile and a ventriculo–peritoneal shunt was inserted at eight weeks of age.

Following surgery there was a sharp fall in haemoglobin and a repeat scan showed a large clot in the occipital horn of the right ventricle (arrows) (**4**). Although the initial clotting screen was reported as normal, repeat clotting studies showed a factor V deficiency after her second bleed.

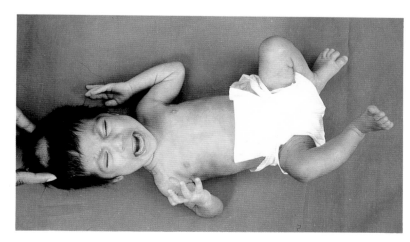

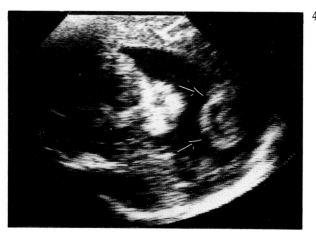

Three shunt revisions were necessary during the first nine months. Her head circumference continued to grow along the 10th centile (**5**).

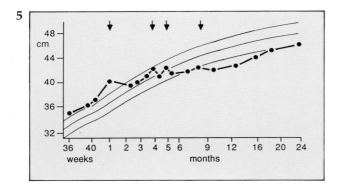

5

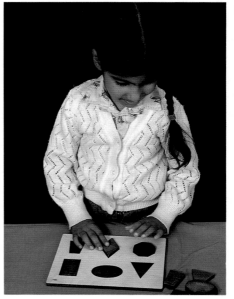

6

Clinical examination: At birth she was jittery, but no other abnormality was found. However, by two weeks of age she had become abnormal, with very poor head control and poor visual pursuit and alertness. At six months she looked alert but did not appear to follow any objects. Abnormal eye movements and a squint were seen at this time. She had marked head lag but otherwise her tone was normal. There were no asymmetries. During the next few months her squint became more pronounced but her vision improved. At one year of age she had some motor delay, was hypotonic, but showed no other neurological abnormalities. She walked at 18 months, she had a persistent squint, and minimal asymmetry of tone in her legs. These signs were still present at four years of age (**6**). She was able to build a tower of nine bricks (**7**) and cope with puzzles (**8**) appropriate for her age.

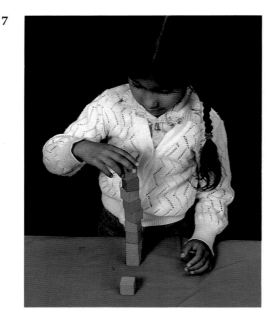

7

8

Magnetic Resonance Imaging: The inversion recovery scan at 40 weeks postmenstrual age showed an extracerebral blood clot (arrows) and asymmetry in ventricular size, with a large right occipital porencephalic cyst (**9**). Low signal intensity areas (dark) were present in the periventricular regions.

At 18 months of age the ventricles had decreased in size, but the right occipital porencephalic cyst was still present, causing midline shift (**10**). There was less myelin posteriorly than anteriorly.

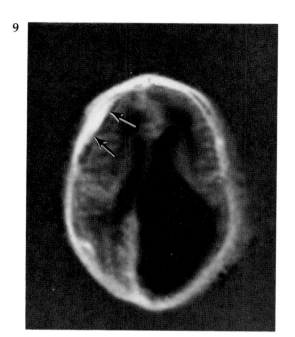

9

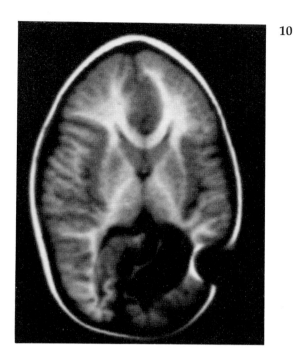

10

Comment: This case illustrates that an important brain lesion may be picked up accidentally. It is of interest that this infant appeared normal following delivery. It is unlikely that a diagnosis of an antenatal insult would have been made if the first scan had been done when the child required shunt insertion at eight weeks of age. It appears to be worthwhile to perform clotting studies in full term infants who show large intracranial lesions at birth. These may be related to intraventricular or intracranial haemorrhage which may have occurred several weeks earlier. The poor visual function in this child is probably related to the bilateral occipital involvement with porencephaly on the right and pressure by the cyst on the left.

Case 2

Preterm infant born at 36 weeks gestation. Her mother fell down the stairs four weeks before delivery, and an antenatal ultrasound scan showed a subdural haematoma (**11**). The child appeared well following an elective caesarean section (**12**). Clotting studies showed a factor X deficiency. She was treated with weekly infusions of factor IX concentrate, until she died following a cerebral haemorrhage at nine months.

11

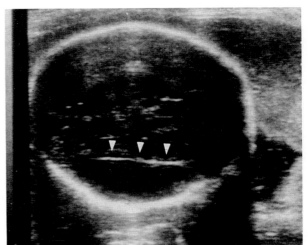

12

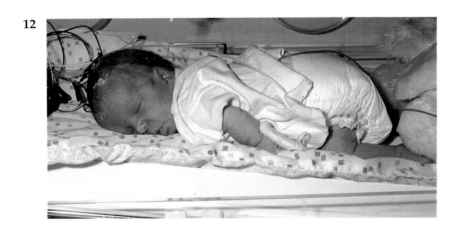

Electroencephalogram: Continuous 4-channel EEG recording on day 1 showed discontinuity and marked asymmetry (**13**).

13

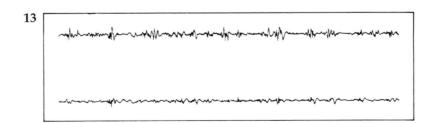

Ultrasound confirmed the diagnosis of a left subdural haematoma, and the left ventricle appeared compressed (**14**). There was a marked shift of the interhemispheric fissure (**15**), and above the cerebellum a cystic lesion was seen in the sagittal midline view (**16**) (arrow). After the clotting deficiency had been corrected, 30 mls of heavily blood-stained fluid was removed by a subdural tap.

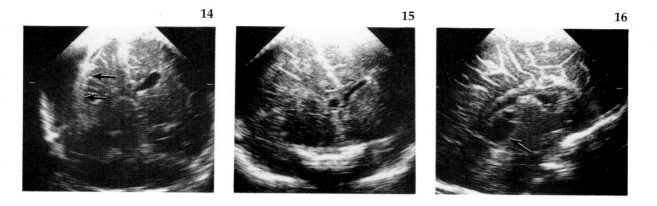

X-ray Computed Tomography (CT): The subdural haematoma was seen as an area of decreased attenuation on the left (**17**), with compression of the left lateral ventricle. An area of low attenuation was visible at the low ventricular level (**18**) and the posterior horn of the right ventricle was dilated.

Magnetic Resonance Imaging (MRI): On day 6 an extensive left subdural haematoma and a smaller right haematoma were seen as high signal intensity areas on the inversion recovery sequence. This appearance indicated that the haemorrhage had occurred between one and four weeks previously (**19**).

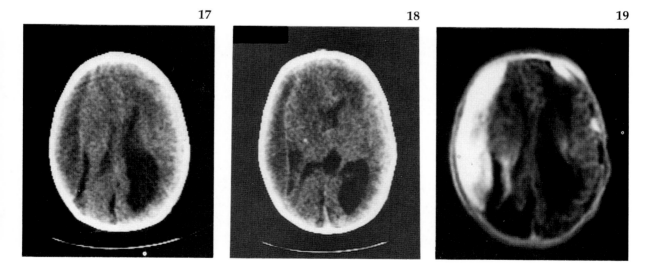

At six weeks of age there was a reduction in the size of the subdural collections at the low ventricular level on the inversion recovery scan (**20**). Areas of low signal intensity were seen in the periventricular regions (arrows).

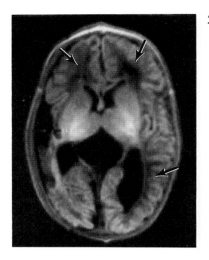

Clinical examination: At six months of age the child was bright and alert (**21**). The only abnormalities were a right adducted thumb, and a slight asymmetry in tone, which was found on careful neurological examination.

On the **CT** scan at nine months of age, there was a large intracerebral haemorrhage occupying much of the left frontal lobe. There was an associated mass effect with displacement of the brain stem (**22**).

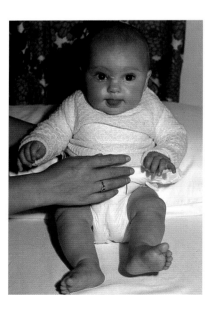

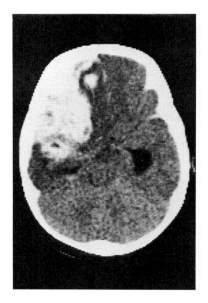

Comment: This case illustrates that even relatively slight maternal trauma may be associated with intracranial lesions; coagulopathy could be held responsible in this particular case.

Convexity lesions may easily be missed using ultrasonography, but, as the lesion was extensive, it was possible to confirm the diagnosis made antenatally. It is of interest that MRI not only showed the extent of the subdural haematoma better than either CT or ultrasound, but was also of help in identifying the time of onset of the haemorrhage.

Case 3

Premature infant with allo-immune thrombocytopenia. Sequential ultrasound studies were performed during pregnancy and an intracranial haemorrhage was seen at 35 weeks gestation. An intravascular platelet transfusion was carried out under ultrasound guidance and the infant was delivered by an elective caesarean section. At six months of age he was cortically blind and showed signs of cerebral palsy.

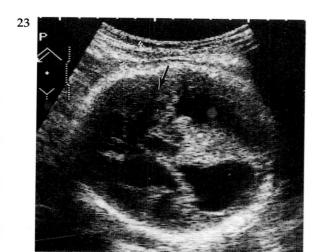

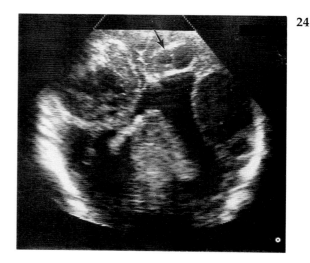

Ultrasound: The antenatal scan performed immediately before delivery showed a left anterior haematoma and dilated ventricles (arrow) (**23**). The postnatal ultrasound scan on day 1 showed several lesions. In the coronal plane, with the scan head angled backwards, a large echolucent area was seen in the right hemisphere (arrow), and a partly echodense area in the left hemisphere (arrow). The ventricles were dilated. Small periventricular cystic lesions were also seen around the right ventricle (arrow) (**24**). The right parasagittal view showed a large cystic area behind the occipital horn of the lateral ventricle (arrow), and multiple periventricular cysts in the fronto–parietal region (arrow) (**25**).

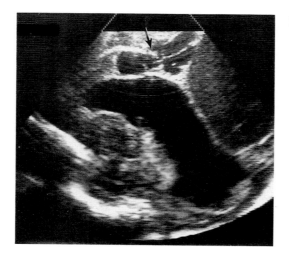

A **CT** scan on day 11 showed the two cystic areas seen on ultrasound and also a third, smaller, cystic area in the left hemisphere and a subarachnoid haemorrhage. The attenuation was slightly increased in the left frontal cystic lesion suggestive of haemorrhage. The periventricular cysts seen on ultrasound were not identified (**26**). The ventricles were enlarged, especially the posterior horn on the left.

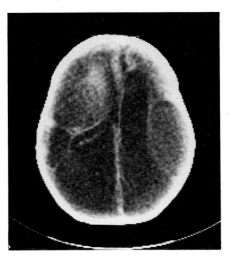

26

Magnetic Resonance Imaging: On day 5 a subarachnoid haemorrhage was seen as high signal intensity on the inversion recovery scan (**27**). There was bilateral ventricular dilatation, which was more marked in the posterior horn of the left lateral ventricle. A subacute haemorrhage, with a rim of high signal intensity and a central core of low signal intensity, was seen anteriorly in the left hemisphere (arrow). The area of low signal intensity (arrows) in the right hemisphere was consistent with chronic haemorrhage. The partial saturation sequence at the same level showed low signal intensity areas at the margins of the haematomas, and in the interhemispheric fissure (arrows) (**28**), and an increased signal intensity (bright) in the chronic haemorrhage. The low signal areas seen on this sequence are the breakdown products of haemorrhage, such as methaemoglobin and haemosiderin.

27

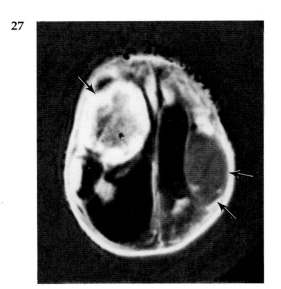

28

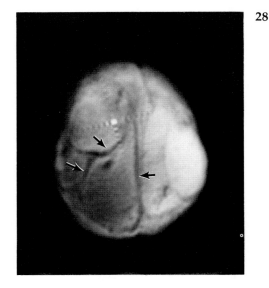

Electroencephalogram: Continuous 4-channel EEG at the end of the first week was severely abnormal with excessive discontinuity, low amplitude and asynchrony (**29**).

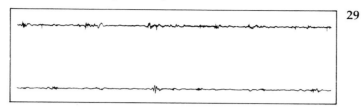

29

On **clinical examination** soon after birth, the infant had extended posture of the legs with increased flexion of the arms (**30**). Hypotonia and marked head lag were seen as the infant was pulled to sit (**31**). A close-up of the baby's hand shows an adducted thumb and a flexed forefinger (**32**). These findings are common in children with cystic leukomalacia, but not in infants with haemorrhage.

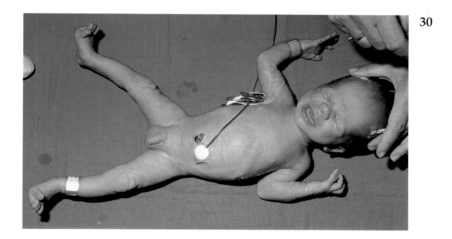

30

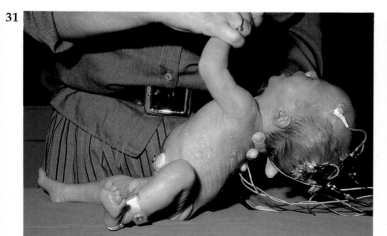

31

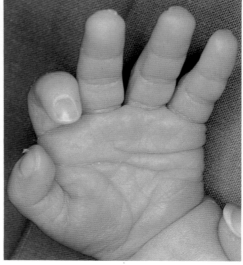

32

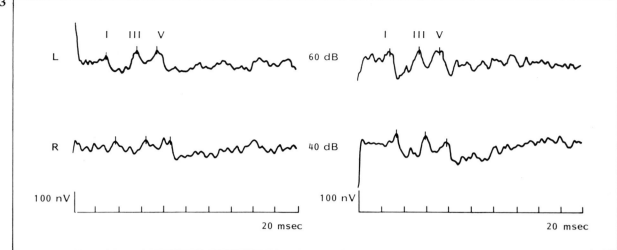

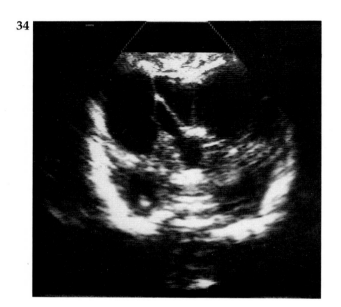

Visual Evoked Responses: No adequate responses were elicited.

Auditory Brainstem Evoked Response: At 36 weeks, responses were apparent, but the response was less clear on the left, particularly at 40 dB (**33**).

At six months, septi were identified on ultrasound, and the echolucent areas were in communication with the ventricles (**34**).

Magnetic Resonance Imaging: The inversion recovery scan at six months showed marked ventricular dilatation and a left frontal porencephalic cyst. An area of low signal intensity (arrow) was seen in the right hemisphere separate from the ventricles. No myelin was identified (**35**). The susceptibility map showed phase changes in the regions of the previous haemorrhage (arrows) (**36**).

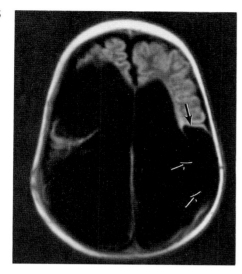

35

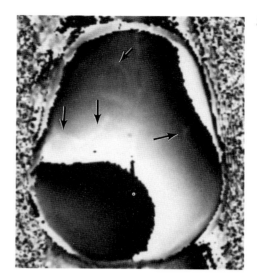

36

Clinical examination: At six months he was extremely irritable, and therefore difficult to assess. There was increased extensor tone of the legs when he was held in a standing position (**37**). His head circumference had exceeded the 97th centile, the intracranial pressure was raised, and the child could not follow. He tended to fall backwards from the sitting position unless held forwards (**38**), and he had spontaneously extending big toes.

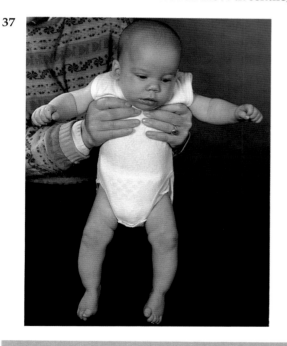

37

38

Comment: This infant developed large parenchymal haemorrhages on several occasions between 30 and 34 weeks gestation. It is of interest that cystic leukomalacia was present as well at the time of delivery. It is likely that cerebral hypoperfusion occurred following severe blood loss. The absence of periventricular leukomalacia in case 1 may have been due to the difference in maturity at the onset of the lesions. The cystic lesions were again best seen on ultrasound. However, ultrasound did not show the extent of the convexity haemorrhage; this was better shown on CT and MRI. MRI was particularly helpful as it showed that there had been several bleeds at different times, demonstrating the extent of the resolving haemorrhages more clearly.

Case 4

Premature infant born at 34 weeks gestation with a birth weight of 1160 grams (<3rd centile). Loss of beat to beat variability, and type 2 dips, were noted on the cardiotocogram several days before delivery, and the infant was delivered by caesarean section. Ventilation for transient tachypnoea was required between 24 and 48 hours. At nine months of age he was a bright, responsive infant with a hemiplegia involving the arm more than the leg.

Ultrasound on day 1 showed small cysts adjacent to the right occipital horn and an irregularly dilated right occipital horn (**39** and **40**). The area around the cyst became much more echodense on the second day and thus the cyst could no longer be identified.

The small cysts seen with **ultrasound** on day 1 became more obvious and extensive at the end of the first week of life, as shown in the coronal and parasagittal views (**41** and **42**).

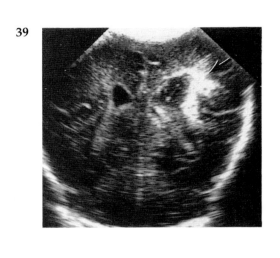

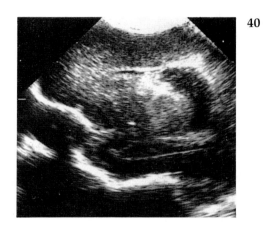

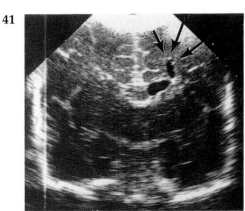

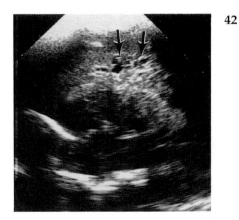

Electroencephalogram: Continuous 4-channel EEG was normal, except for excessive discontinuity during the first week of life (**43**).

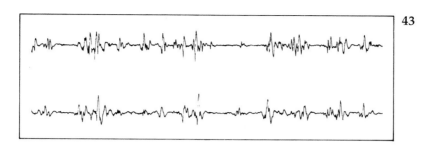

43

Clinical examination at four weeks showed several deviant neurological signs. He had normal leg flexion, but increased arm flexion in the supine position (**44**). When pulled to sit, he had marked head lag (**45**).

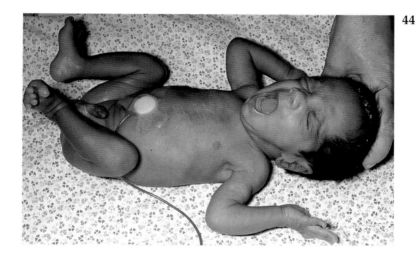

44

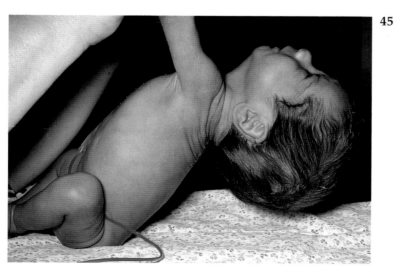

45

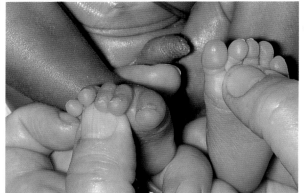

There was asymmetry in tone and his plantar grasp was poor on the left (**46**). Lying on his back at four months he was extremely irritable and showed leg extension with spontaneous up-going toes (**47**). When held in a sitting position, he tended to keep his hands fisted and throw himself backwards (**48**). At nine months of age he had improved greatly and could sit with slight support (**49**). He preferred to use his right hand and tended to keep his left hand fisted (**50**).

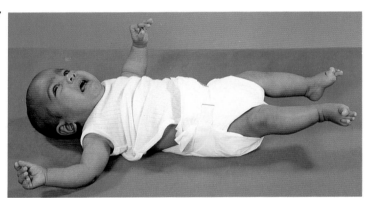

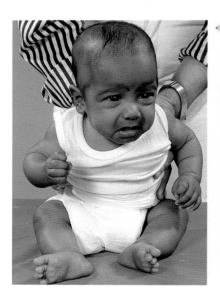

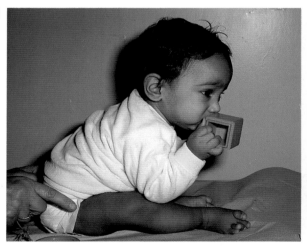

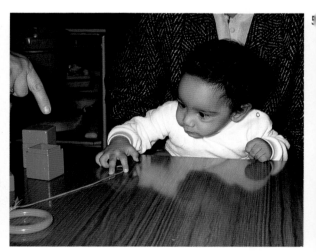

There was no asymmetry of his popliteal angles (**51**), but both toes were still up.

Magnetic Resonance Imaging: At 42 weeks postmenstrual age there was evidence of haemorrhage in both thalami, but it was much more extensive on the right.

At 10 months, ventricular dilatation was seen which was greater on the right than on the left. Myelin was delayed in the left hemisphere and little myelin was seen in the right hemisphere. The remnants of the haemorrhage were seen as high signal intensity on the inversion recovery sequence (arrows) (**52**), and as low signal intensity on the partial saturation sequence (**53**) (arrows).

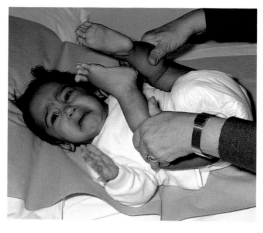

51

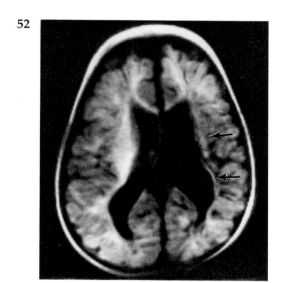

52

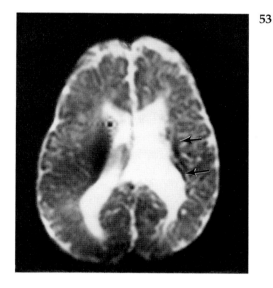

53

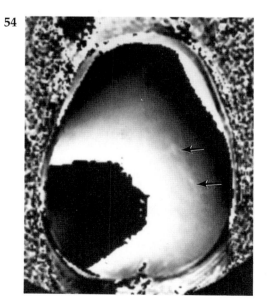

54

The susceptibility map showed phase differences in the same regions (arrows) (**54**).

Comment: This infant was severely compromised antenatally and developed intracranial lesions before delivery. It was not possible to be certain about the true nature of these lesions; it might have been an antenatal intraventricular haemorrhage with associated unilateral periventricular leukomalacia, or an antenatal haemorrhagic infarct.

The fact that the EEG was normal shortly following delivery also supports the antenatal onset of the lesion.

Case 5

Premature infant born at 32 weeks gestation, with a birth weight of 1900 grams. An elective caesarean section was done for pre-eclamptic toxaemia. No problems occurred in the neo-natal period (**55**). There was evidence of periventricular leukomalacia at birth and she subsequently developed cerebral palsy with developmental delay.

55

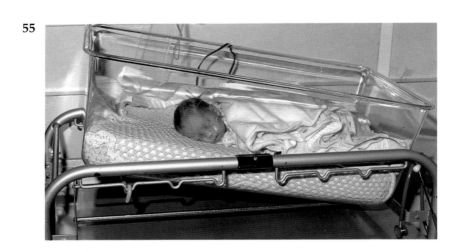

Ultrasound: a coronal view on day 1 showed marked echogenic areas at the external angles of the anterior horns of the lateral ventricles. A small cyst was also present on the right (arrow) (**56**). Ten days later, extensive cystic lesions were seen which extended quite far out from the ventricles, especially on the right (arrows) (**57**). On the parasagittal view cysts were present in the trigone (arrows), but not around the occipital horns (**58**).

56　　　　　　57　　　　　　58

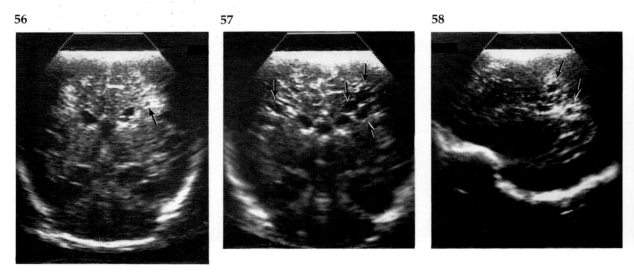

Clinical examination: At 40 weeks postmenstrual age there was poor flexion of the legs but increased flexion of the arms in the supine position (**59**). She had marked head lag when pulled to sit (**60**). In ventral suspension her trunk control was normal but there was a tendency for her legs to hang down (**61**).

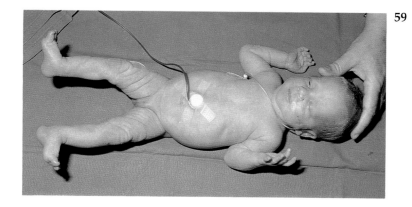

59

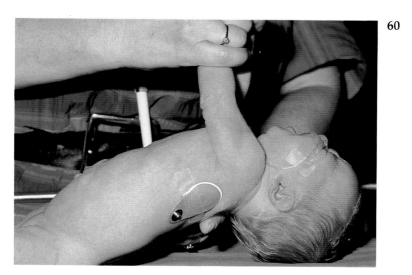

60

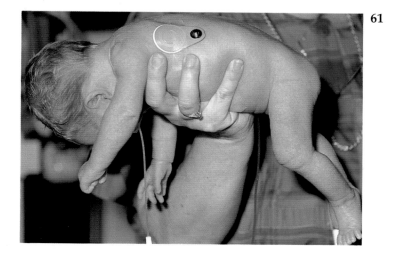

61

At six months she was alert and sociable, and was able to roll on her side and reach out to grasp a ring (**62**). She could keep her head in line with her body when pulled to sit (**63**), and sat with support (**64**). The popliteal angles were tight (**65**). At nine months the tone pattern had changed, the child was hypotonic and still unable to sit without support (**66**).

62

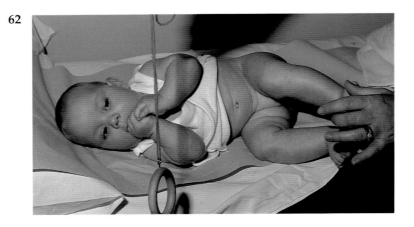

63

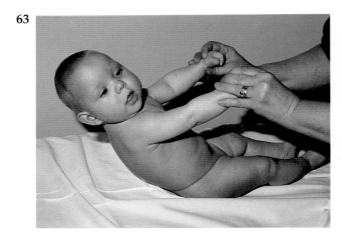

64

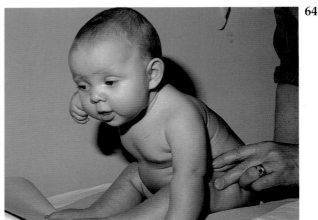

65

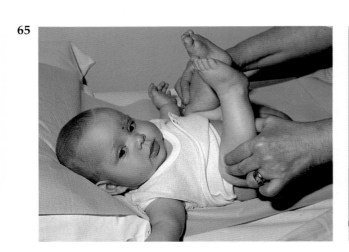

66

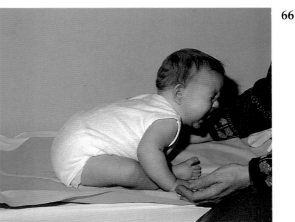

There had been only slight progression in her developmental milestones. Her head circumference had dropped below the third centile. At 15 months of age some progress had been made. She was able to play with boxes and remove the lids (67), and sat without support for a short period (68), but she was unable to bear her weight properly (69). She still had marked tightness of the popliteal angles (70). At 18 months she was unable to stand unaided and she performed at about a 10-month level on the Griffiths scale.

67

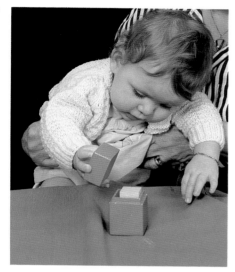

68

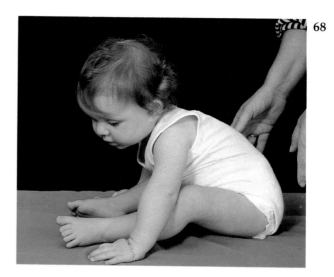

69

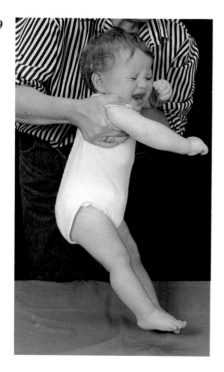

70

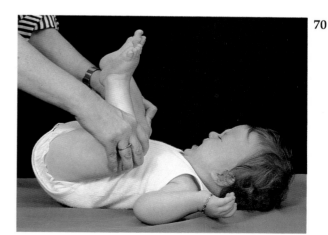

Magnetic Resonance Imaging: On the inversion recovery scan at nine months the ventricles were slightly dilated and irregular posteriorly. Myelination was delayed, especially posteriorly (**71**). High signal intensity areas (arrows) were seen anteriorly on the short TI inversion recovery sequence at a mid-ventricular level, and the ventricles were dilated more anteriorly than posteriorly (**72**).

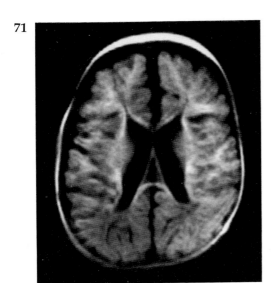

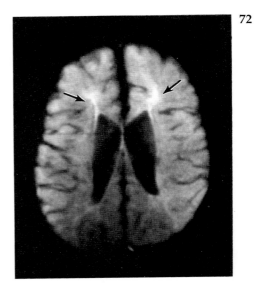

Comment: In this case it is likely that the time of onset of the periventricular leukomalacia was before delivery, as cysts were seen on the first day of life. The neonatal course of this infant was completely uneventful. This case stresses the importance of routinely scanning all admissions and not only those weighing 1500g or less.

It is of interest that there was also some mental impairment in this infant with only anterior lesions, although she did not develop infantile spasms.

Case 6

Premature infant born at 33 weeks gestation. Her co-twin died *in utero* at 29 weeks gestation. The child appeared well, but a multicystic encephalomalacia was seen on routine ultrasound scanning. She developed severe quadriplegia.

Ultrasound: A mid-coronal view showed mild ventricular dilatation and a cystic area above the right ventricle (**73**) (arrow). With the scan head angled backwards, two very large cystic lesions were seen (**74**). On the right parasagittal view the small anterior cyst and the large occipital cyst were separate from the lateral ventricle (**75**).

At three months of age, the **CT** scan showed large occipital cystic lesions (**76**).

73
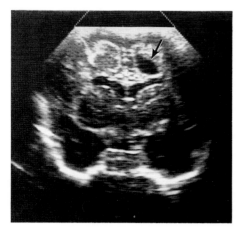

74
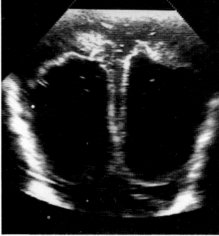

75
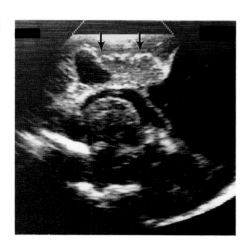

76
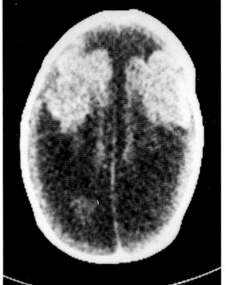

Visual Evoked Responses at 40 weeks postmenstrual age were present despite the large occipital cystic lesions (**77**).

Clinical examination: At 38 weeks postmenstrual age she showed marked flexion of her arms and a flexed posture of her right forefinger (**78**). At five months of age her posture was still remarkably normal in ventral suspension (**79**). At nine months, however, she was extremely hypertonic and tended to lie in an opisthotonic posture (**80**). She could, however, focus and follow a red ball (**81**).

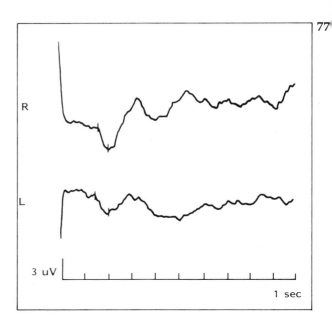

77

R

L

3 uV

1 sec

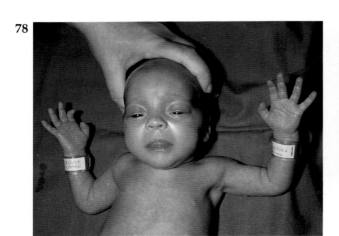

78

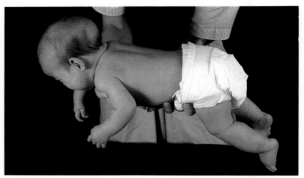

79

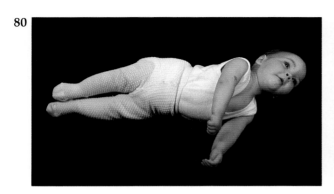

80

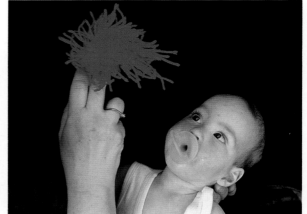

81

Magnetic Resonance Imaging: Scans were done at six and 18 months of age. An inversion recovery scan at mid-ventricular level showed large areas of low signal intensity in the occipital regions at six months (**82**). There was cortical atrophy and the ventricles were enlarged, and no myelin could be identified (**82**). Bilateral shunts were inserted into the occipital cysts at 15 months. At 18 months, the ventricles had increased in size, whereas the occipital cysts had decreased in size (**83**). Myelin was seen around the anterior horns of the lateral ventricles. A corresponding short TI inversion recovery sequence showed areas of high signal intensity in the periventricular regions which were more marked posteriorly (arrows) (**84**).

82
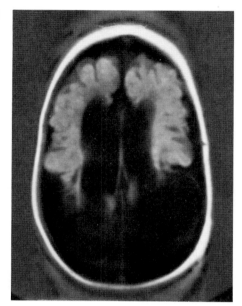

83
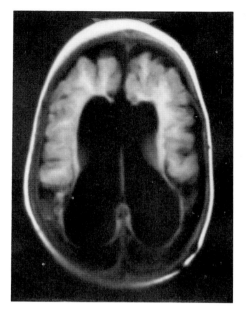

84
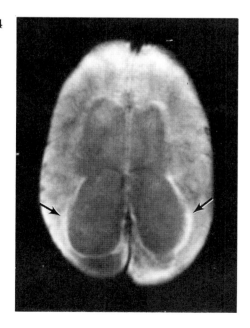

Comment: This case stresses the importance of performing an ultrasound scan at birth, when there is a history of a macerated co-twin. This should be done even, as in this case, when the surviving twin appears to be perfectly well at birth (even at five months the child showed few grossly abnormal signs).

It is of interest that this child retained her vision despite bilateral occipital lesions.

Chapter 6. Hypoxic Ischaemic Encephalopathy in the Full Term Infant

Pathological Features

A variety of lesions can be identified on histological examination. The most important are: (i) selective neuronal necrosis; (ii) parasagittal cerebral injury; and (iii) status marmoratus.

Clinical Recognition

Cranial **ultrasound** is not as useful and reliable here as it is in haemorrhage or leukomalacia. The presence of increased echogenicity and loss of normal anatomical structures is often, but not always, related to the presence of cerebral oedema.

An **X-ray Computed Tomography (CT)** scan may be helpful in these infants, and should be done if **Magnetic Resonance Imaging** is not available. MRI is more sensitive to haemorrhage and changes in the basal ganglia, and in the periventricular regions. MRI would also be the imaging method of choice for the long-term follow-up.

Doppler studies can provide additional information, as a low Pulsatility Index (<0.55) is strongly related to a poor outcome.

A full **clinical examination** is important. According to Sarnat, the infants can be divided into three groups according to the presence of: (a) hyperalertness and hyperexcitability; (b) hypotonia and suppressed primitive reflexes; or (c) stupor, flaccidity and the absence of primitive reflexes.

In addition, seizures and neurological abnormalities which are slow to resolve are useful in identifying the infants who are most at risk for later sequelae.

Electrophysiological Tests

Auditory Brainstem Evoked Response can be completely normal in severely affected children with a poor outcome. Abnormalities in wave shape and amplitude may be present and an abnormal wave V:I ratio has been reported to be of predictive value.

Visual Evoked Response can be of predictive value in infants who develop severe visual impairment. Absence of, or very poor and inconsistent, responses are usually found during the neonatal period.

Electroencephalogram (EEG): The EEG has been extensively documented as one of the most sensitive guides to outcome in asphyxiated term infants. The state of the background EEG activity is more predictive than the presence of seizure discharges. Normal background activity correlates strongly with normal outcome and severe depression with later major neurological sequelae. With background abnormalities of intermediate severity, the rate of resolution is the best guide to prognosis. Continuous 4-channel EEG is also extremely useful for monitoring the effectiveness of treatment in seizure control.

Case Histories

Case 1

This was the second of twins, delivered at 40 weeks by ventouse extraction, 80 minutes after the first twin. At birth she was pale, and hypotensive with bradycardia. Despite immediate intubation, her Apgar scores were 2, 4, 5 and 7 at one, five, 10 and 20 minutes respectively. Regular respirations were only established at 22 minutes and she required ventilation until eight hours of age. Following initial hypotonia, she became hypertonic with an extended posture (1) at a few hours of age. A loading dose of phenobarbitone (20 mg/kg) was given at 10 hours for excessive 'rowing movements' and irritability. Several convulsions were noted during the second day of life, which responded to intramuscular paraldehyde. A subarachnoid catheter was inserted at 34 hours of age and a raised pressure of 26mmHg was recorded with a cerebral perfusion pressure of 30mmHg. After the administration of Mannitol the intracranial pressure fell to 18mmHg (normal <6mmHg). Her neurological status deteriorated further and she died at 96 hours of age.

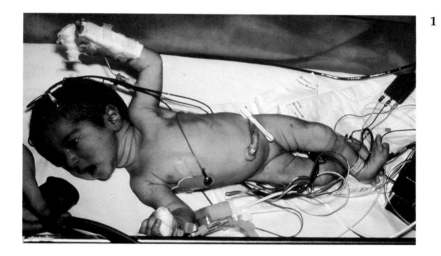

Electroencephalogram on the second day of life was severely abnormal, with persistent seizures on an asymmetrical low amplitude background, which deteriorated to the isoelectric state in the following days (2).

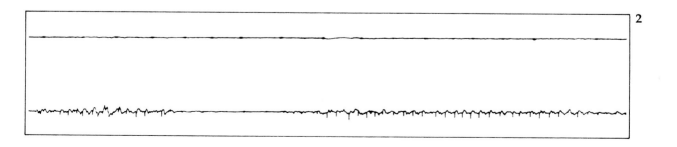

169

Ultrasound examinations on the first day of life were normal (**3**). On day 3 there was a diffuse increase in echogenicity and a loss of normal anatomy (**4**).

3
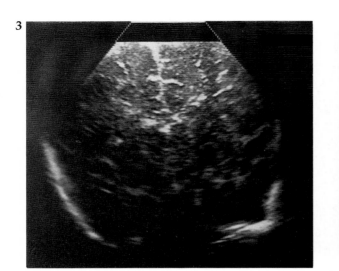

4
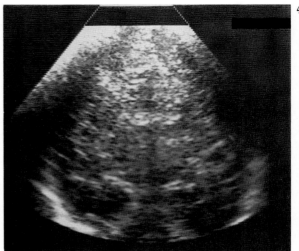

Auditory Brainstem Evoked Responses on day 3 showed good responses at 80 and 60 dB on the left. On the right there was an abnormal wave V:I ratio at 80 dB, but this was not present at 60 dB (**5**).

5
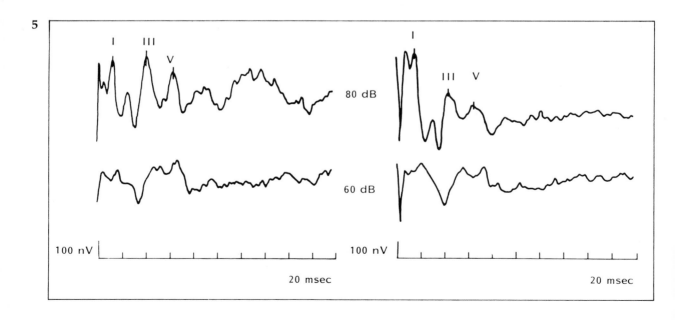

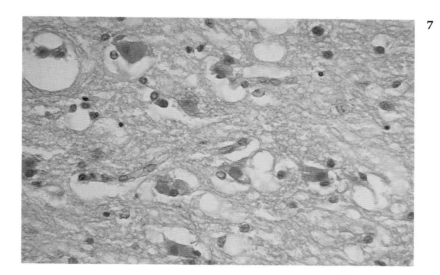

At **autopsy** the brain was swollen and oedematous, with flattened convolutions. Coronal sections after fixation revealed compressed ventricles but no focal lesions (**6**).

On histological examination there was severe anoxic–ischaemic damage involving all areas of the cerebrum including cortex, white matter, thalamus and hippocampus. In addition, changes were seen in the mid-brain, pons, dentate nucleus and medulla. Coagulative necrosis of the neurones of the thalamus is shown in **7** (Haematoxylin and Eosin × 250).

Comment: This case illustrates that, in a severely asphyxiated infant, abnormal ultrasound appearances may not be present until two to three days of age. The EEG, however, tends to be abnormal from day 1. In this case the increased echogenicity seen on the ultrasound scan was associated with a raised intracranial pressure. However, the ABR was within normal limits despite the raised intracranial pressure and the serious general condition of the child.

The following five cases reflect the variety of outcome which can be seen in term infants with birth
asphyxia.

Case 2

Male infant born at 39 weeks gestation. Meconium stained liquor and type II dips on the cardiotocograph were noted to precede delivery. The child was eventually delivered by an emergency caesarean section, following failed ventouse and forceps extraction. Apgar scores were 0, 2 and 7 at one, five and 10 minutes respectively. Regular respirations were present at 14 minutes of age when he was successfully extubated. At six hours of age generalised convulsions occurred which were treated with a loading dose of phenobarbitone and three doses of intramuscular paraldehyde.

The infant was referred to our unit at 10 days of age. At the time of referral the ultrasound scans were normal.

8

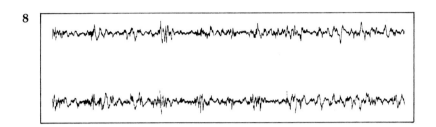

Electroencephalogram: Continuous 4-channel EEG recorded following admission showed normal amplitude and continuity with some bilateral sharp waves (8).

A **CT** scan performed on day 15 was suggestive of decreased attenuation in the periventricular regions (9 and 10).

9

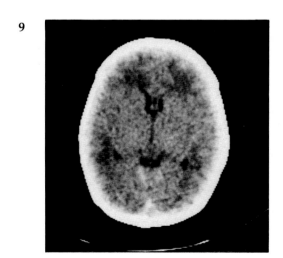

10

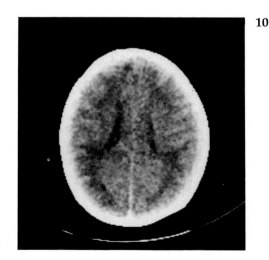

Clinical examination: A right lower motor neurone facial palsy was noted (**11**). He had bilateral fisted hands and adducted thumbs, but a normal posture in the supine position (**12**). His posture was also normal in ventral suspension (**13**), but he had marked head lag when pulled to sit (**14**). At 10 months of age his development was normal. He sat well without support (**15**), and could stand with slight support (**16**). Slight hypotonia was still present. At 18 months he was neurologically normal.

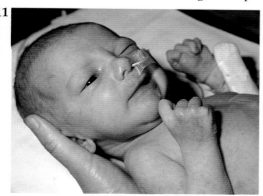

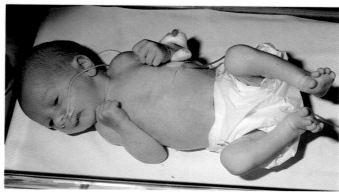

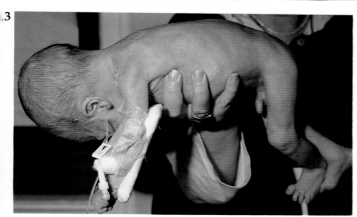

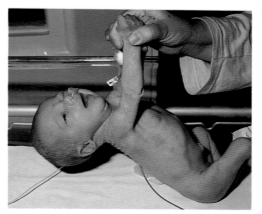

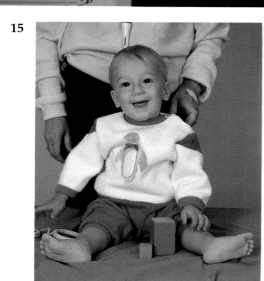

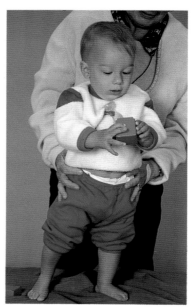

Magnetic Resonance Imaging: At two weeks of age the inversion recovery sequence showed low signal intensity areas in the periventricular regions and high signal intensity in the basal ganglia (arrows) (**17**). On the corresponding partial saturation sequence, low signal intensity was seen in the basal ganglia (arrows) (**18**). These findings were suggestive of haemorrhage. The inversion recovery scan at low ventricular level at 13 months showed myelination within normal limits (**19**), although the white matter in the thalami had a higher signal intensity than white matter in the rest of the brain. There were still areas of low signal intensity in the basal ganglia on the partial saturation sequence, but these were less marked than in the neonatal period (**20**).

17

18

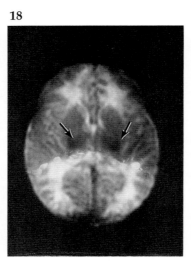

19

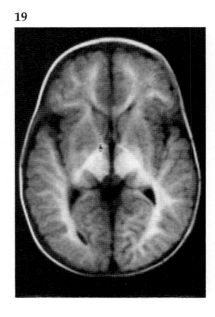

20

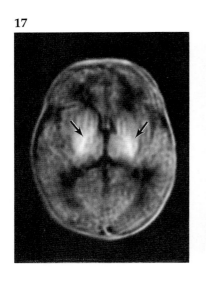

Comment: This case illustrates that it is more difficult to give an accurate prognosis when imaging studies and electrophysiological tests cannot be performed during the first week of life, and when the rate of clinical recovery is not well documented. Both the ultrasound and CT scans were normal at the time of referral, but both may have shown lesions beforehand. Magnetic resonance imaging is helpful, since it may show abnormalities for a longer time. The signal intensity on both sequences was consistent with blood in the basal ganglia. However, no permanent neurological deficit occurred despite this finding. This case also shows that severely asphyxiated infants may have a normal outcome even when some abnormal neurological signs persist beyond the first week of life.

Case 3

Male infant born at 39 weeks gestation by spontaneous vaginal delivery. A foetal heart rate of 100/min was recorded for twenty minutes before delivery and the cord was drawn tightly around his neck. Apgar scores were 1 and 3 at one and five minutes respectively. The child was intubated immediately, and the heart rate picked up but he remained limp. His first regular respirations were at 20 minutes of age and he was extubated at 25 minutes. He suffered a prolonged convulsion at six hours. He remained tremulous and irritable for two weeks, but improved considerably over the next few weeks. His tone pattern was definitely abnormal at five months. Athetoid cerebral palsy was diagnosed in his first year of life.

Electroencephalogram: Continuous 4-channel EEG recording on the second day showed severe abnormalities (**21**). The amplitude was low and there was extreme discontinuity. There was marked asymmetry with a greater depression on the right than on the left. Frequent sharp waves were seen on the left.

Ultrasound examinations were unremarkable. Minimal periventricular echogenicity was seen on day 2, but the anatomical structures were easily identified (**22**). At 10 days mild ventricular dilatation was present (**23**).

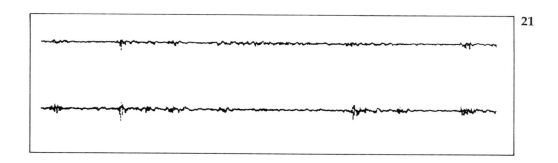

21

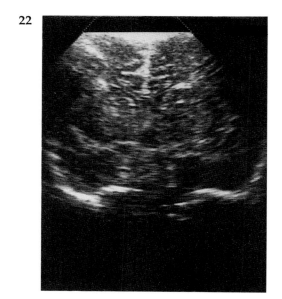

22

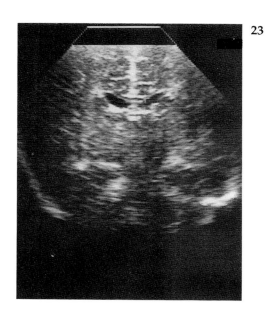

23

A **CT** scan on day 11 suggested decreased attenuation in the periventricular regions (**24**).

Magnetic Resonance Imaging: The inversion recovery sequence on day 9 showed patchy areas of high signal intensity in the region of the basal ganglia (arrows) consistent with haemorrhage (**25**), and low signal intensity in the periventricular regions (arrows).

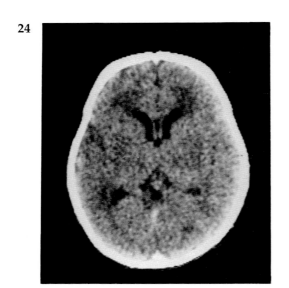

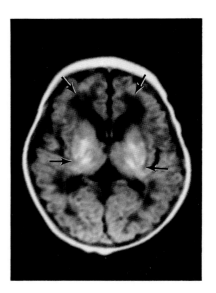

Auditory Brainstem Evoked Responses: On day 7 the responses were present at 80 and 60 dB intensity, but wave V was poor and the V:I ratio was abnormal (**26**).

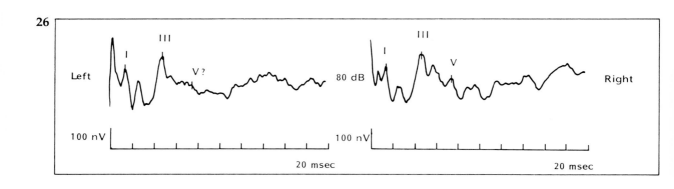

Clinical examination: He was very tremulous and irritable during the first two weeks but there was considerable improvement by two months. However, although less irritable, he remained tremulous and had increased flexor hypertonia.

At five months he had an abnormal tone pattern and very tight popliteal angles. At seven months he showed severe neurological abnormalities. When he was held in a standing position his head posture was abnormal, his hands were fisted and he drooled excessively (**27**). At 18 months of age there was still a marked tightness of his popliteal angles (**28**). However, in ventral suspension he showed trunk hypotonia and he was unable to elevate his legs (**29**). His lateral tilting reactions were absent (**30**).

27

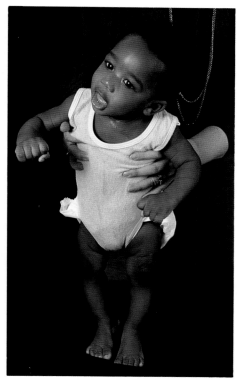

28

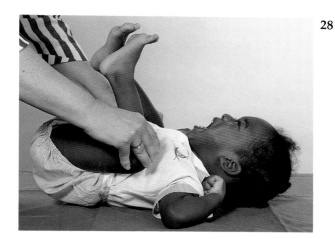

29

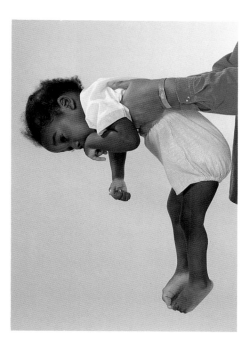

30

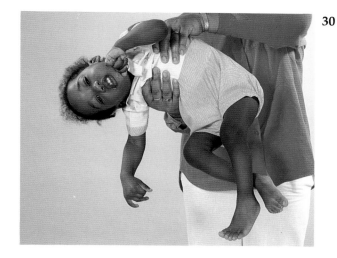

He was bright and, despite his severe motor disabilities, he managed to pick up objects from the table (**31**).

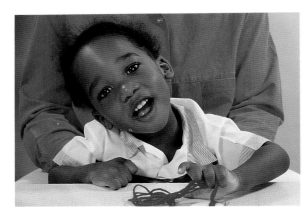

Magnetic Resonance Imaging: The inversion recovery scan at 22 months of age showed myelination at the expected level for his age and low signal intensity ·areas in the posterior lentiform nuclei (arrows) (**32**). These lesions were seen as high signal intensity areas on the short TI inversion recovery sequence (arrows) (**33**).

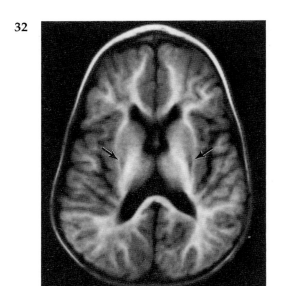

32

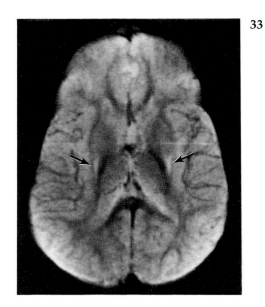

33

Comment: This case illustrates the limited information obtained using cranial ultrasound in a term infant who subsequently develops athetoid cerebral palsy. On CT the lesion in the basal ganglia was not very striking. As the CT scan was not done until day 11 it is possible that there had been a haemorrhage and the blood had become isodense. MRI showed the lesions in the basal ganglia, which, in contrast to case 2, figures **19** and **20** (page 174), were more obvious at 18 months.

Note that his clinical abnormalities, especially his tremulousness, persisted far beyond the neonatal period.

Case 4

Female infant born at 40 weeks gestation by an emergency caesarean section for foetal distress. Apgar scores were 0 and 5 at one and five minutes respectively. She was intubated, and regular breathing started at 15 minutes of age. She was extubated at 20 minutes and no further ventilation was required. Her first convulsions were apparent at 24 hours, and these convulsions were seen inter-mittently for three days. She was given a loading dose of phenobarbitone. At follow-up at nine months she was alert, with abnormal tone pattern but no definite signs of athetoid cerebral palsy.

Ultrasound: On day 2 a diffuse increase in echo-genicity was seen (34), with a loss of anatomical definition. Two days later, anatomical structures were recognisable and there were bright bands in both thalami (35).

34
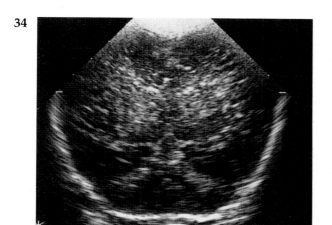

35
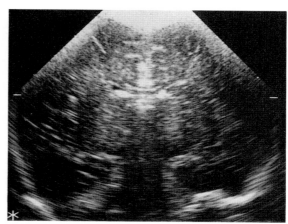

Electroencephalogram: Continuous 4-channel EEG done on day 1 showed excessive discontinu-ity, frequent sharp waves, and seizure activity (arrow) (36).

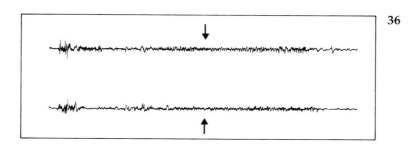

36

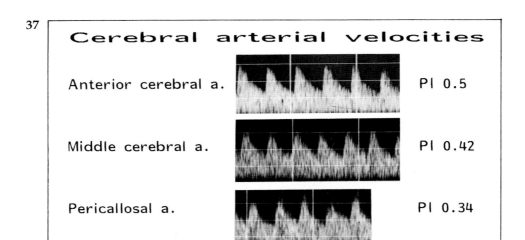

Cerebral arterial velocities

Anterior cerebral a.   PI 0.5

Middle cerebral a.   PI 0.42

Pericallosal a.   PI 0.34

Doppler studies: Using pulsed Doppler, the middle and anterior cerebral arteries were located and the pulsatility index was persistently below 0.55 over a period of two to three days (**37**).

A **CT** scan done at three days of age was unremarkable (**38**).

Magnetic Resonance Imaging: On day 10 the inversion recovery scan showed areas of high signal intensity in the basal ganglia (arrows) (**39**), and low signal intensity in the periventricular regions.

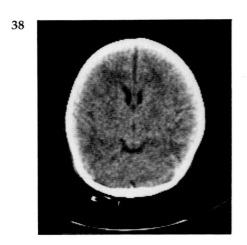

38

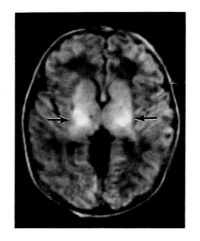

39

Clinical examination: During the first few days of life she remained almost motionless, with marked arm flexion and some leg extension (**40**). Flexion of the legs occurred when the head was brought forward (**41**), and marked head lag was present when she was pulled to sit (**42**). At three months of age she was still hypertonic and extremely irritable, and no visual following could be obtained. She had increased extensor tone in the trunk and flexor tone in the limbs. She was unable to fix her pelvis when pulled to a sitting position (**43**), and she showed marked arm flexion and neck extension when held in a sitting position (**44**). She had severe feeding difficulties at this age.

40
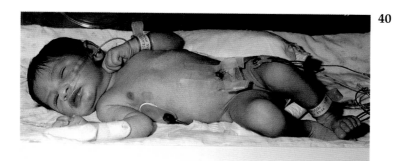

41
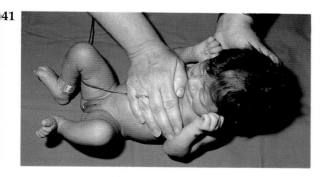

42
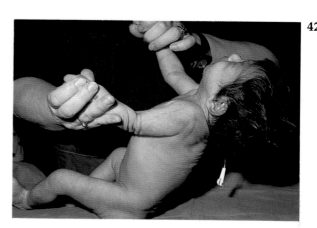

43
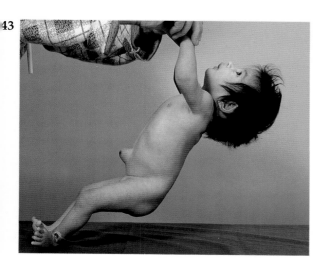

44
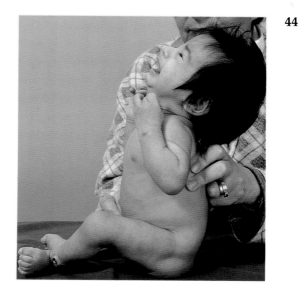

At nine months of age she still had a variable tone pattern with tight popliteal angles. She was able to stand with support but was unable to keep her head upright (**45**). Although feeding was difficult, she did not show definite signs of athetoid cerebral palsy.

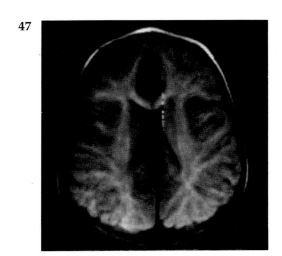

45

Her head circumference had fallen below the 3rd centile by the end of the first month (**46**). However, it was in proportion to her length and weight, and all three parameters continued to increase below, but parallel to, the 3rd centile.

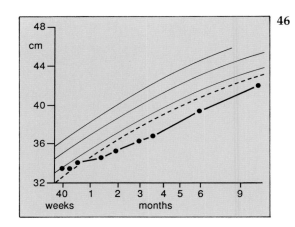

46

Magnetic Resonance Imaging: The inversion recovery scan at nine months of age showed myelination within normal limits at the mid-ventricular level **47**. At the level of the centrum semiovale the myelin was decreased posteriorly, and less myelin was seen in the left hemisphere **48**.

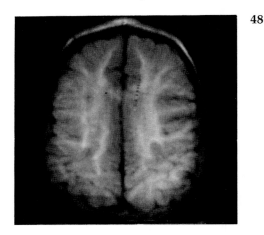

47

48

Comment: This case once again illustrates the limited information obtained using ultrasound and CT scans in infants with birth asphyxia. The first MRI examination suggested the presence of blood in the basal ganglia, but she is still too young for it to be certain that she will develop athetoid cerebral palsy.

The EEG and Doppler studies were particularly useful. The importance of the EEG in infants with birth asphyxia in relation to prognosis, especially the background activity, has been appreciated for a long time. The low pulsatility index seen in asphyxiated infants (<0.55) has been reported by Levene *et al* to be a strong predictive value for a poor outcome.

On clinical examination, as in the previous case, abnormal neurological signs persisted beyond the neonatal period.

Case 5

Male infant born at 40 weeks gestation by caesarean section because of foetal distress. Type II dips and meconium stained liquor were noted an hour and a half before delivery. Apgar scores were 3 and 6 at one and five minutes respectively. Regular respirations were present at eight minutes after face mask ventilation. A loading dose of phenobarbitone was given at one hour of age. Frequent convulsions were noted from 12 hours of age which were difficult to suppress. After transfer he was electively hyperventilated during the first four days of life. The intracranial pressure measured with a subarachnoid catheter was raised (15mmHg), but the cerebral perfusion pressure was satisfactory.

Electroencephalogram: 4-channel EEG on admission showed a burst suppression pattern with frequent seizures (**49**) (arrows).

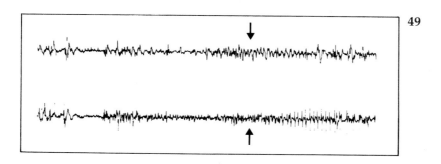

49

Ultrasound examination on day 4 showed a diffuse increase in echogenicity and a loss of anatomical structures (**50**).

A **CT** scan done on day 11 showed blood in the region of the heads of the caudate nuclei (arrows) (**51**).

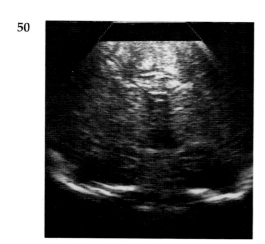

50

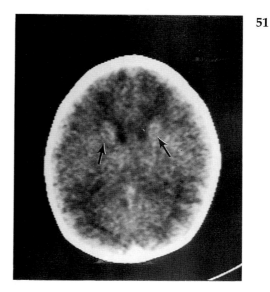

51

Clinical examination: He was hypotonic during the first few days, with less movement on the left. Asymmetry was less marked by day 9. At two weeks he was irritable, and there was a slight increase in extensor tone. At two months he appeared clinically normal except for a slight tightness of the popliteal angle on the right. However, at six months of age he had signs of a hemiplegia, which was still marked at 18 months (**52**). His head circumference was on the 3rd centile at birth, and fell below the 3rd centile at two months of age (**53**). At 20 months he developed seizures for which he received regular treatment. At three years of age his hemiplegia was less marked, but his intellectual deficit was more obvious.

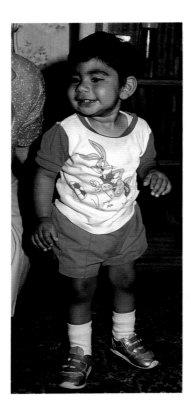

52

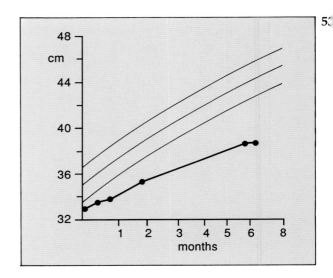

53

Magnetic Resonance Imaging: The inversion recovery sequence at seven days showed high signal intensity in the thalami suggestive of haemorrhage (arrows) (**54**).

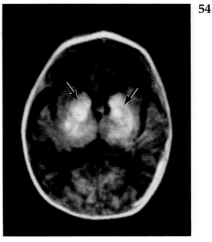

54

At 26 months of age, myelination was within normal limits anteriorly and laterally, and there was a mild delay posteriorly (**55**). The short TI inversion recovery sequence showed high signal intensity in the choroid plexus (arrows) (**56**). This is a common finding, the significance of which is uncertain.

55

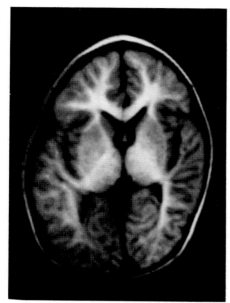

56

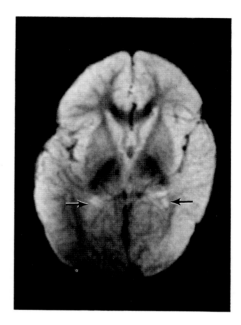

Comment: Ultrasound showed diffuse increased echogenicity and loss of anatomical structures. These findings have been reported to be associated with cerebral oedema, and the intracranial pressure was indeed raised in this infant.

The thalamic haemorrhages were not seen with ultrasound, but were shown on CT and MRI. These haemorrhages were the most remarkable feature in the neonatal period; however, they did not have any specific sequelae as in case 3. The reason for the hemiplegia in this child remains unclear.

Again, the EEG was the best early predictor for later problems. In this case, in spite of a very quick clinical recovery, he did not have a normal outcome.

Case 6

Full term infant delivered at 42 weeks gestation. Meconium stained liquor was seen for nine hours before delivery. Apgar scores were 3 and 9 at one and five minutes respectively. Intubation was performed at two minutes of age. Extubation was not tolerated and ventilation was required for the first four days. Seizures were frequent and persisted for three days.

The child developed severe cortical atrophy and was quadriplegic and microcephalic, with severe visual impairment, at 12 months of age.

Continuous 4-channel EEG was severely ab-normal for a prolonged period, with seizure activity on a low amplitude background.

Ultrasound performed on day 2 showed a diffuse increase in echogenicity and a loss of anatomical structures (**57**). Pulsations were poor in the middle and posterior cerebral artery, and absent in the anterior cerebral artery. Intracranial pressure measured with a subarachnoid catheter was normal. Two weeks later, ventricular dilatation and widening of the interhemispheric fissure occurred. Severe cortical atrophy was seen at four months (**58**).

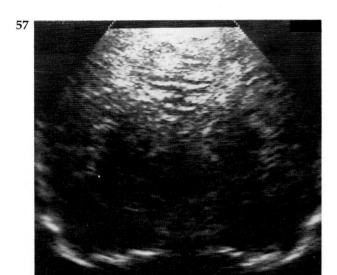

57

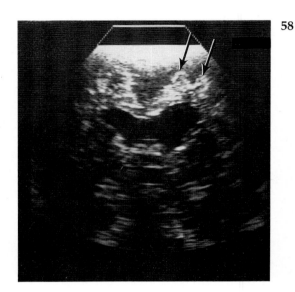

58

A **CT** scan on day 19 showed increased attenuation in the basal ganglia and thalami (**59**).

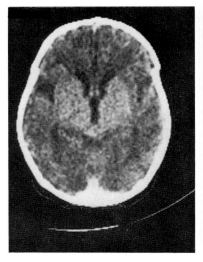

59

Auditory Brainstem Evoked Responses at six days of age were normal with a threshold of 20 dB intensity (**60**).

Visual Evoked Responses: No responses could be elicited during the neonatal period.

Clinical examination: On the initial examination, the infant was unresponsive and severely hypotonic. At three weeks of age he had improved and was able to follow a red woollen object (**61**). He was hypotonic in a supine position, with abducted legs and adducted thumbs (**62**). Marked head lag was present when pulled to sit (**63**).

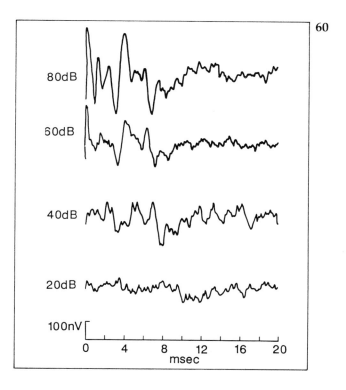

60

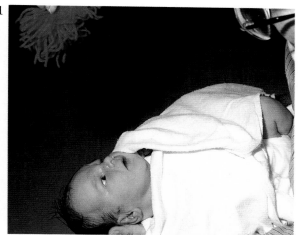

61

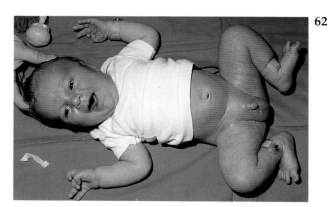

62

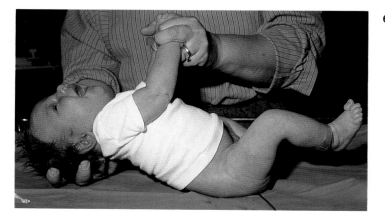

63

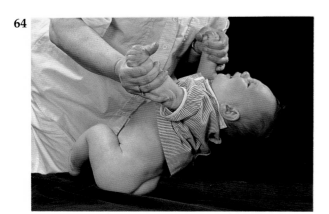

64

At four months the head lag persisted (**64**). In ventral suspension his legs hung down when his head was above the plane of his body (**65**). There was increased extensor tone of the legs with scissoring and internal rotation of the arm (**66**). He was microcephalic (**67**). Cortical blindness was suspected at this stage and his visual evoked responses were still absent (**68**).

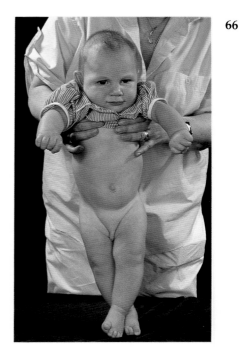

66

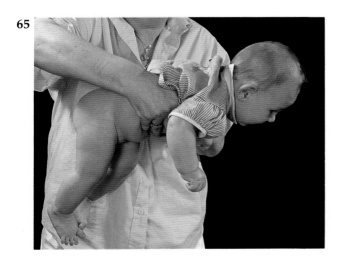

65

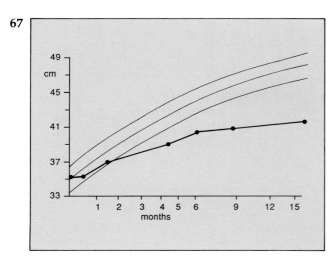

67

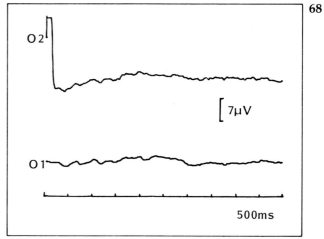

68

At nine months his vision was still in doubt but some visual evoked potentials could be elicited in the temporal region (**69**). By 18 months visual responses were also present in the occipital region (**70**).

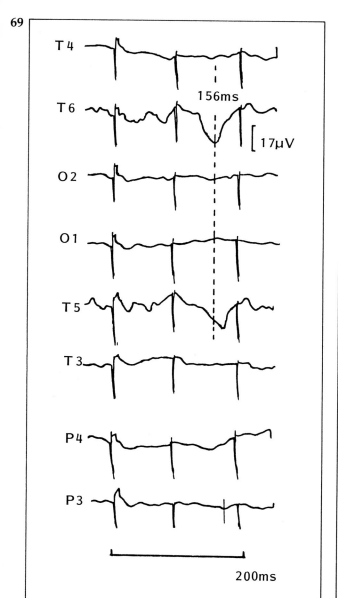

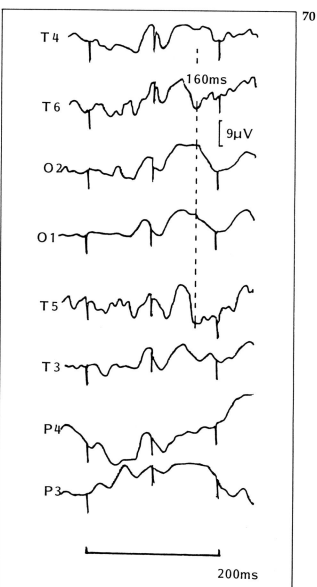

Clinically, at 9 months, there was a slight improvement in visual function (**71**). He was unable to sit without support (**72**), and when held to stand his posture had changed little since five months of age (**73**; cf **66**).

71

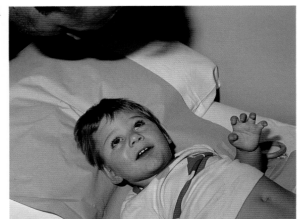

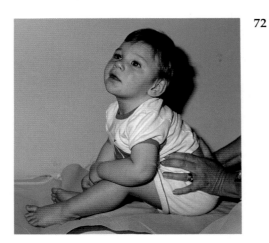

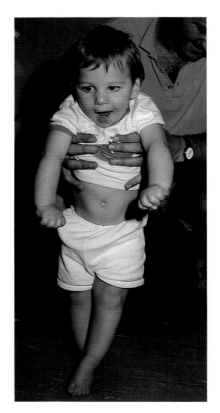

Magnetic Resonance Imaging: The inversion recovery scan at four weeks of age was degraded by movement artefact, but areas of high signal intensity were seen in the region of the basal ganglia. At 15 months there was ventricular dilatation, especially in the occipital horns, and cortical atrophy was seen. Myelination was severely delayed (**74**). The partial saturation sequence (**75**) showed low signal intensity in the basal ganglia (arrows), which corresponded with the high signal intensity in **74**. These findings and the pattern of high signal seen at four weeks of age indicated that a haemorrhage in the basal ganglia had occurred during the perinatal period.

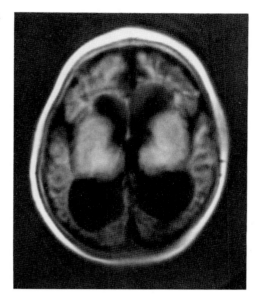

74

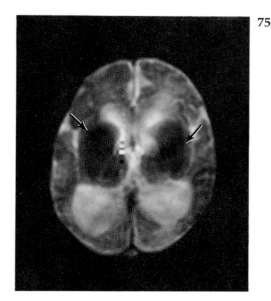

75

Comment: Ultrasound showed loss of anatomical structures and a diffuse increase in echogenicity. In contrast to the previous case, the intracranial pressure was normal. In spite of the similar initial ultrasound appearance, the clinical development in this child was very different from the previous case and marked cortical atrophy developed.

MRI showed the most extensive changes, particularly in the basal ganglia, and these changes persisted beyond the neonatal period. The exact nature of these lesions is not certain and status marmoratus was considered. It is of interest, however, that, in spite of these extensive changes in the basal ganglia, there was no evidence of athetoid cerebral palsy.

The EEG was a good early predictor, and severe abnormalities were present for a long period.

On clinical examination, deviant neurological signs persisted far beyond the neonatal period, again suggesting a poor outcome.

Case 7

Female infant born at 42 weeks gestation by a vaginal vertex delivery. Meconium stained liquor was present. Her Apgar scores were 3 and 6 at one and five minutes respectively. The baby was tachypnoeic, and developed dusky spells associated with convulsions at eight hours of age. A diagnosis of persistent foetal circulation was made, but she maintained adequate pO2 levels without mechanical ventilation. Her convulsions were treated with phenobarbitone and later with diazepam. At four years of age there was no gross motor impairment, but she was very clumsy. She also exhibited a severe sensorineural hearing loss and mild to moderate mental retardation.

Ultrasound: On the second day of life a localised area of increased echogenicity was seen behind the occipital horns of the lateral ventricles (**76**).

A **CT** scan on day 7 showed extensive areas of decreased attenuation throughout both hemispheres; this was most marked in the occipital regions (**77**).

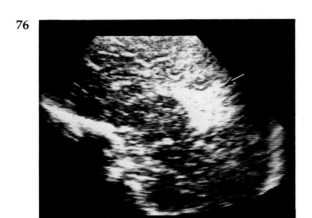

76

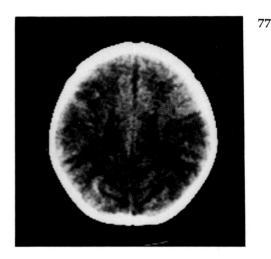

77

Clinical examination: She had persistent abnormal neurological signs in the neonatal period and her development was abnormal at three months. Her posture was abnormal in ventral suspension with internal rotation of her arms (**78**), and there was marked tightness of her popliteal angles (**79**). She developed seizures at nine months, for which she received regular treatment.

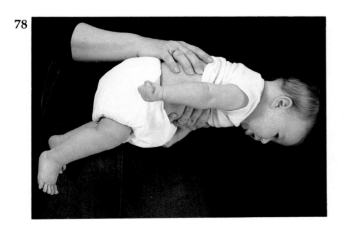

78

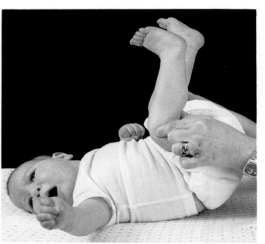

79

Her motor development improved considerably and by two years of age she walked unaided (**80**). She had relatively good auditory brainstem responses in the neonatal period, but at two years she had sensorineural deafness and there was some degree of mental retardation. At four years of age she attended a school for deaf children, she was short sighted and rather clumsy, but had no major motor deficit.

Magnetic Resonance Imaging: Inversion recovery scans at low ventricular level and through the centrum semiovale are shown at 10 months of age. The ventricles were slightly enlarged, especially posteriorly, and the occipital poles were atrophied. Myelin was delayed posteriorly but within normal limits anteriorly (**81**). At the level of the centrum semiovale there was marked local cortical atrophy posteriorly, and low signal intensity areas were seen in both occipital poles (arrows) (**82**).

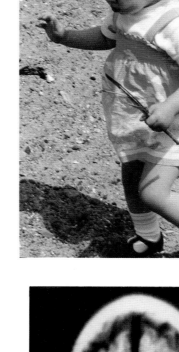

80

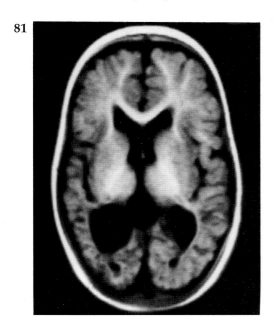

81

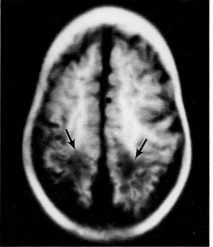

82

Comment: The abnormalities seen with ultrasound, CT and MRI are different from those in the previous six cases. Marked abnormalities were seen in the occipital regions. On ultrasound, localised areas of increased echogenicity were seen around the occipital horns of the lateral ventricles. In our experience this finding is uncommon in infants with birth asphyxia, but it has been described by Volpe as a parasagittal watershed injury. The ultrasound studies did not show the extensive diffuse cortical involvement, which was visible on the neonatal CT and the later MRI scans. Despite the marked occipital involvement, no visual problems occurred until three years of age, when her shortsightedness was diagnosed. The cause of the later sensorineural deafness is not clear, but cytomegalo virus infection could possibly account for it; however, her viral studies were negative. Another point of interest is that her early abnormal motor pattern did not relate to any major motor abnormalities later on.

Principles of Magnetic Resonance Imaging: Glossary, References and Suggested Reading

Glossary

Field gradient: a magnetic field which changes in strength in a certain direction. Such fields are used in MRI to select the slice and spatially encode the signal. Gradient magnetic fields are measured in *Teslas* per metre.

Fourier transformation: a mathematical procedure to separate out the frequency components of a signal from its amplitudes as a function of time, or vice versa. The Fourier transformation is used to generate the spectrum from the FID in pulsed nuclear magnetic resonance (NMR) techniques, and is essential to most imaging techniques.

Free induction decay (FID): after a 90° pulse a transient NMR signal will result which decays towards zero with a characteristic time constant (T2): this decaying signal is the FID.

Inversion recovery sequences (IR): this sequence uses a 180° radiofrequency pulse followed at a time TI later by a 90° pulse, and is usually employed to produce images in which the contrast is mainly dependent on the differences in T_1 (medium TI form), although image contrast is also influenced by proton density and T_2.

Inversion time (TI): the time between the 180° and the subsequent 90° pulse to elicit an NMR signal in inversion recovery.

Main static magnetic field: the principal magnetic field which aligns nuclear spins in the same direction.

MHz: megahertz, million cycles/second.

Magnetic susceptibility: the ability of a substance to become magnetised. There are three types – diamagnetism, paramagnetism and ferromagnetism.

Partial saturation sequence (PS): this sequence uses a 90° pulse repeated at TR intervals. Data collection uses a field echo rather than a spin echo. Contrast in these images is dependent on proton density, T_1, T_2, chemical shift and susceptibility effects.

Proton density: the number of hydrogen nuclei per unit volume.

Pulse sequence: a series of short magnetic field pulses rotating at the nuclear spin frequency (i.e. radiofrequency for protons) which are used to rotate the patient's proton magnetisation through 90° or 180°. The commonly used examples are partial saturation, spin echo and inversion recovery. The names are derived from classical nuclear magnetic resonance spectroscopy.

Receiver coil: a tuned radiofrequency coil which picks up the NMR signal.

Signal-to-noise ratio: used to describe the relative contributions to the detected signal of the true signal and random superimposed signals ('noise').

Spin echo sequence (SE): this sequence uses a 90° pulse followed at time TE/2 later by a 180° pulse. Data are collected when an echo of the original signal is obtained at time TE later. This sequence produces images whose contrast mainly reflects differences in T_1 and T_2. The contrast in a spin echo sequence with short TR and TE is mainly dependent on T_1 relaxation and is known as a T_1 weighted image. A spin echo sequence with a long TR and TE is mainly T_2 dependent and is termed a T_2 weighted sequence.

Tesla: the SI unit of magnetic flux density. One *tesla* is equal to 10,000 gauss, the older (CGS) unit.

Transmitter: portion of the NMR apparatus that produces radiofrequency current and delivers it to the transmitting coil.

T_1 relaxation time (spin lattice relaxation time): spin lattice or longitudinal relaxation time; the characteristic time constant for spins to tend to align themselves with the main static magnetic field. Starting from zero, magnetisation in the z direction, the z magnetisation, will grow to 63% of its final maximum value in a time T_1.

T_2 relaxation time: spin-spin or transverse relaxation time: the characteristic time constant for loss of phase coherence among spins oriented at an angle to the static magnetic field, due to interactions between the spins, with resulting loss of transverse magnetisation and NMR signal. Starting from a non-zero value of the magnetisation in the xy plane the xy magnetisation will decay so that it loses 63% of its initial value in a time T2.

TE (echo time): the time between the 90° pulse and data collection in a Partial Saturation, spin echo or inversion recovery sequence.

TI (inversion time): Time after the inverting 180° radiofrequency pulse to the middle of the 90° pulse in an inversion recovery sequence.

TR (repetition time): The period of time between the beginning of a pulse sequence and the next cycle.

References

1. Dubowitz LMS, Pennock JM, Johnson MA, Bydder GM. High resolution magnetic resonance imaging of the brain in children. *Clinical Radiology*, 1986;37;113–117.
2. National Radiological Protection Board *ad hoc* Advisory Group on Nuclear Magnetic Resonance Clinical Imaging. Revised guidance on acceptable limits of exposure during nuclear magnetic clinical imaging. *British Journal of Radiology*, 1983;56;974–977.
3. Yakovlev PI, Lecours AR. The myelogenetic cycles of regional maturation in the brain. In: Minkowski A, ed. *Regional development of the brain in early life*. Oxford: Blackwell Scientific, 1967 pp 3–69.
4. Johnson MA, Pennock JM, Bydder GM *et al*. Clinical NMR imaging of the brain in children: normal and neurological disease. *American Journal of Neuroradiology*, 1983;4;1013–1026, and *American Journal of Radiology*, 1983;141;1005–1018.
5. Johnson MA, Pennock JM, Bydder GM *et al*. Serial Magnetic Imaging in neonatal cerebral injury. *American Journal of Neuroradiology*, 1987;8;83–92.

Suggested Reading

Gadian DG. *Nuclear magnetic resonance and its applications to living systems*. Clarendon Press, Oxford, 1982.
Stark DD and Bradley WG (eds). *Magnetic Resonance Imaging*. CV Mosby, St Louis, 1988.

Index

All references are to page numbers

A

Aberrant signs 12
Abnormal movement/posture 9
Alertness 10
Allo-immune thrombocytopenia, infant
    with 151
Amnionitis 45
Anterior cerebral artery velocity 180
Arm recoil 9
Arm release in prone position 9
Arm traction 9
Auditory brainstem evolved responses 14-15
- cerebral artery infarction 135
- haemorrhagic/ischaemic lesions, antenatal
    154
- hypoxic ischaemia 168, 170, 176, 187
- intraventricular/ periventricular
    haemorrhage 32, 38, 49, 54, 67
- leukomalacia 72
- - periventricular cystic 97
- - subcortical 121, 126
Auditory orientation 10

B

Birth asphyxia 182
- increased echogenicity around occipital
    horns 193
- low pulsatility index 182
Brainstem transmission time 14

C

Cardiotocogram recordings 144, 156
Cerebral artery infarction (neonatal stroke)
    135-143
- auditory brainstem evoked responses 135
- case histories 136-143
- clinical recognition 135
- CT scan 136, 140, 142
- electroencephalogram 135, 136
- haemorrhagic infarct 141
- hemiplegia 143
- historical background 135
- magnetic resonance imaging 137, 139, 141,
    143
- non-haemorrhagic lesion 141
- pathological features 135
- premature/term infants compared 143
- ultrasound 136, 140, 142
- visual evoked responses 135
Cerebral arterial velocities
- anterior cerebral artery 180
- middle cerebral artery 18, 180
- pericallosal artery 180
Cerebral oedema 185
Cerebral palsy 43, 113
- athetoid 178
- post-periventricular leukomalacia 108-111
- see also Spastic diplegia
Chloral hydrate 23
Clinical evaluation 8-13
- scoring chart 9-10
Clotting studies 147
Computed tomography (CT)
- cerebral artery infarction 137, 140, 142
- haemorrhagic/ischaemic lesions, antenatal
    149, 150, 152
- hypoxic ischaemia 168, 176, 178, 180, 183,
    185, 186, 192
- intraventricular/periventricular
    haemorrhage 30, 33, 42
- leukomalacia 70
- - mixed cystic 112
- - periventricular cystic 102, 103
- - subcortical 121
Consolability 10
Co-twin, macerated 165, 167
Cry 10
Cytomegalovirus infection 193

D

Defensive reaction 10
Development
- aberrant signs 12
- delayed 12
Doppler ultrasound 18

- haemorrhagic/ischaemic lesions, antenatal 144
- hypoxic ischaemia 168, 180

E
Electroencephalography 15-17
- cerebral artery infarction 135, 136
- haemorrhagic/ischaemic lesions, antenatal 153, 157
- hypoxic ischaemia 168, 169, 172, 175, 179, 183, 185, 186, 191
- intraventricular/periventricular haemorrhage 32, 33, 35, 64
- leukomalacia 72, 74
- - mixed cystic 116
- - periventricular cystic 92, 94
- - subcortical 125, 127
- prognostic indicator 17
Electrophysiology 14-17
- auditory brainstem evoked responses 14-15
- electroencephalography 15-17
- somatosensory evoked responses 15
- visual evoked responses 14-15
Eye appearances 10

F
Factor X deficiency 148
Finger posture abnormality 13

G
Gastroschisis 120
Germinal layer haemorrhage 33

H
Habituation
- light 9
- rattle 9
Haemorrhagic/ischaemic lesions of antenatal origin 5, 144-167
- auditory brainstem evoked responses 154
- cardiotocogram recordings 144, 156
- case histories 145-167
- causes 144
- cerebral function monitor 144
- clinical examination 144
- CT scan 149, 150, 152
- Doppler studies 144
- electroencephalogram 153, 157
- electrophysiological tests 144
- historical background 144
- magnetic resonance imaging 147, 149, 152, 154, 158, 164, 167
- onset 8
- pathological features 144
- ultrasound 88, 91, 144, 145, 149, 151, 156, 160, 165
- visual evoked responses 154, 166
Head control 9
Head lag 9
Head raising in prone position 9
Hearing assessment 13
Hemiplegia 55, 184
Hyaline membrane disease, infant with 42, 48, 60
Hypoxic ischaemia in the full term infant 168-193
- auditory brainstem evoked responses 168, 170, 176, 187
- case histories 169-193
- clinical examination 168
- coagulative thalamic neuronal necrosis 171
- CT scan 168, 176, 178, 180, 183, 185, 186, 192
- Doppler studies 168, 180
- electroencephalogram 168, 169, 172, 175, 179, 183, 185, 186, 191
- electrophysiological tests 168
- magnetic resonance imaging 168, 174, 176, 178, 180, 184, 185, 191, 193
- pathological features 168
- severely asphyxiated infants 174
- ultrasound 168, 170, 175, 179, 183
- visual evoked responses 168, 187, 189

I
Intraventricular/periventricular haemorrhage 29-68
- asymmetry in tone/movement 30, 44, 45
- auditory brainstem evoked responses 32, 38, 49, 54, 67
- bilateral ischaemic lesions 63
- case histories 33-68
- clinical examination 30
- clinical recognition 29-31
- CT scan 30, 33, 42
- electroencephalogram 32, 33, 35, 64
- germinal layer haemorrhage 33
- hemiplegia 55

- historical background 29
- hypotonia 37, 39, 41
- immature brain 59
- incidence in preterm children 8
- left occipital infarct 57
- magnetic resonance imaging 30, 41, 43, 47, 52, 56, 59, 62-63, 68
- parenchymal haemorrhage 34, 46-47
- parietal lesion 43
- periventricular leukomalacia compared 130-134
- popliteal angle 30
- porencephalic cyst 46, 47, 48, 52, 54, 57
- premature infants 33-64
- progression of clinical signs 30
- somatosensory evoked responses 32
- term infant 65-68
- ultrasound 29, 34, 35, 38, 42, 44, 46, 48, 54, 58, 60, 64, 66
- venous infarction 34
- ventricular dilatation 36, 37
- - measurement by ultrasound 37
- visual evoked responses 32, 39, 49, 58
Irritability 10, 13, 65
Ischaemic lesions of brain 5
- antenatal origin, see Haemorrhagic/ ischaemic lesions

L
Left occipital infarct 57
Leg recoil 9
Leg traction 9
Leukomalacia 69-134
- auditory brainstem evoked responses 72
- case histories: premature infants 73-81
- clinical examination 70-72
- CT scan 70
- cyst formation 77
- electroencephalogram 72, 74
- historical background 69
- magnetic resonance imaging 70, 81
- mixed cystic 69, 80
- - case histories 112-119
- - cortical blindness 112, 115
- - CT scan 112
- - electroencephalogram 116
- - magnetic resonance imaging 115, 118-119
- - mild course 116-119
- - myelination 115
- - ultrasound 112, 116
- - visual evoked responses 113, 117

- onset 8
- pathological features 69
- periventricular cystic 69, 78-79, 81
- - anterior part centrum semiovale 83
- - auditory brainstem evoked responses 97
- - case histories 82, 111
- - CT scan 102, 103
- - electroencephalogram 92, 94
- - haemorrhagic/non-haemorrhagic, ultrasound effect 88, 91
- - infantile spasms associated 84, 87
- - intraventricular haemorrhagic compared 130-134
- - magnetic resonance imaging 83, 86-87, 88, 96, 101, 103, 106-107, 108, 111
- - not diagnosed during early neonatal period 104-111
- - periventricular densities 109
- - posterior part centrum ovale 96
- - ultrasound 82, 84, 88, 92, 94, 97, 103, 104
- - visual evoked responses 97
- selective neuronal necrosis 74
- somatosensory potentials 72
- subcortical cystic 69, 72, 120-129
- - auditory brainstem evoked responses 121, 126
- - case histories 120-129
- - CT scan 121
- - electroencephalogram 125, 127
- - magnetic resonance imaging 124, 128
- - outcome 129
- - visual evoked responses 126
- - ultrasound 120, 125
- transient densities 93
- ultrasound 69, 74, 75, 76-77, 78, 79
- visual evoked responses 72

M
Magnetic resonance imaging 18-28
- cerebral artery infarction 137, 139, 141, 143
- equipment 20-21
- free induction decay 19
- gradient magnetic fields 21
- haemorrhagic/ischaemic lesions, antenatal 147, 149, 152, 154, 158, 164, 167
- hypoxic ischaemia 168, 174, 176, 178, 180, 184, 185, 191, 193
- intraventricular/periventricular haemorrhage 30, 41, 43, 47, 52, 56, 59, 62-63, 68
- leukomalacia 70, 81

-- mixed cystic 115, 118-119
-- periventricular cystic 83, 86-87, 88, 96,
     101, 103, 106-107, 108, 111
-- subcortical 124, 128
- magnetic susceptibility 20
- normal brain appearances 24-27
- pathological brain appearances 27-28
- patient preparation 23-24
- patient safety 23-24
- phenomenon 19
- properties: pulse sequences 22
-- chemical shift 22
-- flow effects 22
-- inversion time 22
-- inversion recovery 22
-- partial saturation 22
-- proton density 21, 22
-- spin echo 22
-- susceptibility 22
-- time to echo 22
-- tissues 21-22
-- T_1/T_2 22
- static magnetic field 19
Maturation
- abnormal 12
- accelerated 12
Maternal trauma 148, 150
Microcephaly 186, 188
Middle cerebral artery velocity 18, 180
Moro response 10

N
Necrotising enterocolitis, infant with 112,
     120
Neonatal stroke, see Cerebral artery
infarction

P
Palmar grasp 10
Peak of excitement 10
Pericallosal velocity 180
Periventricular haemorrhage, see
     Intraventricular/periventricular
     haemorrhage
Placing 10
Plantar grasp 10
Popliteal angle 9
Porencephalic cyst 46, 47, 48, 52-53, 54, 57
Posture 9
- abnormal 9

Preterm infants
- electroencephalography 15
- incidence of intraventricular haemorrhage
     8
- neurological status 8
- overabducted posture of hips 36
- with intraventricular/periventricular
     haemorrhage 33-64
Proton 19
- density 21

R
Raised temperature 65
Respiratory distress syndrome, infant with
     38, 78
Responsiveness 10
Rooting 10

S
Scoring chart 9-10
Sedation 23
Seizures 65
Somatosensory evoked responses 15
- intraventricular/periventricular
     haemorrhage 32
- leukomalacia 72
Spontaneous Babinski 13
Spastic diplegia
- post-periventricular leukomalacia 97, 99,
     104, 110
- transient densities 93
- see also Cerebral palsy
Spontaneous body movement 9
Startles 9
Status mormoratus 168, 191
Subdural haematoma 148-150
Sucking 10
Supine position 11

T
Tendon reflexes 10
Toe posture abnormality 13
Tone pattern, abnormal 13
Transient dystonia, transient densities in 93
Tremors 9

U
Ultrasound imaging 5-11
- cerebral artery infarction 136, 140, 142

- coronal cuts 7
- haemorrhagic/ischaemic lesions, antenatal 88, 91, 144, 145, 149, 151, 156, 160, 165
- hypoxic ischaemia 168, 170, 175, 179, 183
- intraventricular/periventricular haemorrhage 29, 34, 35, 38, 42, 44, 46, 48, 54, 58, 60, 64, 66
- leukomalacia 69, 74, 75, 76-77, 78, 79
-- mixed cystic 112, 116
-- subcortical 120, 125
- parasagittal view 7
- periventricular cystic leukomalacia 82, 84, 88, 92, 94, 97, 103, 104
- sagittal view 7
- sector scanners 6
- standard cuts angles 6
- transient densities 93
- value of repeated scanning 8
- ventricular dilatation measurement 37

V
Venous infarction 34
Ventral suspension 9, 11, 12
Vision assessment 13
Visual evoked responses 14-15
- haemorrhagic/ischaemic lesions, antenatal 154, 166
- hypoxic ischaemia 158, 187, 189
- intraventricular/periventricular haemorrhage 32, 39, 49, 58
- leukomalacia 72
-- mixed cystic 113, 117
-- periventricular 97
-- subcortical 126
Visual orientation 10

W
Walking 10